Nursing care

in Acute Medicine

The complete Guide

ALEXANDRE CAREWELL

Table of contents

« The Acute Medicine Department specialises in the rapid care of patients suffering from sudden illnesses or exacerbations of chronic conditions requiring immediate medical intervention. »

Chapter 1.
INTRODUCTION TO ACUTE MEDICINE

Definition and scope of acute medicine

Acute medicine, often evoked with a certain gravity in hospital corridors, remains at the heart of the medical art. It is concerned with sudden illnesses, abrupt pathologies and physiological disturbances that require rapid, targeted intervention. When a patient arrives at hospital with alarming symptoms, whether sudden chest pain, difficulty breathing or loss of consciousness, they enter the world of acute medicine.

But what does it really mean? Put simply, acute medicine is the branch of medicine dedicated to the immediate assessment and treatment of serious and urgent conditions. It does not stop at one speciality, but encompasses a multitude of disciplines, from trauma to infectious diseases, cardiology and many others. It requires healthcare professionals not only to have an in-depth knowledge of diseases, but also to be able to make informed decisions at times when every second counts.

The scope of acute medicine goes beyond mere medical intervention. It also encompasses the human, organisational and even ethical dimensions of care. Take, for example, a patient who is admitted with respiratory distress: his treatment is not limited to stabilising his breathing. It also includes managing the patient's pain and anxiety, communicating with the family, coordinating with other specialists, and sometimes making delicate decisions about quality of life and end-of-life care.

In the hospital setting, acute medicine is often synonymous with palpable effervescence. Teams move quickly, monitors ring, and health professionals are constantly on the alert, ready to act. But this urgency does not exclude the need for attentive listening, clear communication, and respectful, compassionate care.

Acute medicine is a delicate dance between urgency and patience, between science and humanity. It is a reflection of a fast-moving society, where expectations of care are high and medical technology is constantly evolving. But at the heart of it all remains the very essence of medicine: the unwavering commitment to care, to cure and, when that's not possible, to bring comfort and dignity.

The importance of the nurse in acute care

When one thinks of the busy corridors of an emergency department or the incessant ringing of an intensive care unit, the image that immediately springs to mind is of nurses bustling around beds, connecting patients to monitors, administering medicines and offering soothing words to worried families. At the heart of acute medicine, the nurse plays a pivotal role, often underestimated, but absolutely essential.

Nurses are the true sentinels of acute medicine. They are the first to notice subtle changes in a patient's condition, to intervene when the situation deteriorates and to coordinate care between different healthcare professionals. Their in-depth training enables them to assess clinical situations accurately, initiate vital interventions and provide complex care in complete safety.

But the importance of nurses does not stop at these technical skills. Their role is also intrinsically linked to the human dimension of care. In a medical world where everything seems to speed up, nurses take the time to listen, reassure and educate. They are often the reassuring face that calms worries, the confidant who hears unspoken fears and the guide who clarifies the often complex decisions of patients and their families.

Nurses are also facilitators. In the maze of acute medical care, they act as a link between doctors, therapists, social workers and other team members. They coordinate care, ensure that interventions are carried out in a timely manner and ensure that the care plan is understandable and patient-centred.

They are also the nurses who, day after day, night after night, stand by the patient's bedside, monitoring vital signs, adjusting treatments and providing invaluable emotional support. In moments of crisis, they are the calm in the middle of the storm, skilfully balancing the urgency of the situation with a patient-centred approach.

The impact of nursing on patient outcomes in acute medicine is undeniable. Studies have shown that the quality of nursing care is directly linked to reductions in mortality, complications and readmissions. So, beyond their visible role, nurses play a fundamental role in optimising patients' health and well-being.
In the complex and demanding world of acute medicine, nurses are an anchor, a driving force and a beacon. Their importance transcends medical care and touches on the very essence of what it means to truly heal, support and care.

The transition from student
to professional nurse in acute medicine

The transition from classroom to clinical reality is one of the most profound and significant leaps a nurse can make. Where studies focus on theory, technical skills and simulated scenarios, the real world of acute medicine offers intense immersion in a world where decisions have immediate and tangible consequences.

The transition from student to professional nurse in acute medicine is similar to a metamorphosis. The novice, armed with knowledge but still hesitant, evolves into a confident professional capable of making informed decisions in often stressful situations.

The ocean of clinical realities

As soon as a young nurse sets foot on an acute medicine ward, he or she is confronted with a whirlwind of activity. Patients need immediate care, monitors are ringing, and the urgency is palpable. Where textbooks offered clear, structured cases, reality presents patients with complex symptoms, stories intertwined with co-morbidities, medication and emotions.

Building trust and competence

A newly qualified nurse's first interventions are often marked by double-checking, a reluctance to ask questions, and a dependence on more experienced colleagues. However, as the days go by, repeated practice and accumulated experience forge their competence and confidence. Actions become more confident, the ability to prioritise is refined, and clinical discernment deepens.

The importance of mentoring

The guidance of senior nurses is crucial in this transition process. They act as role models, offer practical advice, share their experiences and, above all, encourage the new nurse to think critically. Informal or structured mentoring can greatly influence the learning curve of new nurses.

Emotional growth

As well as clinical skills, the transition also encompasses an emotional transformation. Faced with suffering, death or ethical dilemmas, young nurses learn to navigate their own emotions, strike a balance between empathy and professionalism, and manage stress and fatigue.

Integration into the team

Another essential aspect is integration into the multidisciplinary team. Learning to communicate effectively with doctors, therapists, care assistants and other team members is crucial to optimal patient care.

This transition is a journey of learning, discovery and personal and professional growth. While it is undoubtedly marked by challenges, it is also marked by achievements that reinforce a passion for the profession and a commitment to the well-being of patients. And, at the end of this journey, there is a fulfilled, competent nurse who is ready to face the varied challenges of acute medicine with confidence and compassion.

Chapter 2.
THE WORKING ENVIRONMENT

Emergency services : front line of acute medicine

Emergency departments are often compared to the gateways to the medical world. They are the first point of contact for many patients faced with crisis situations, whether an accident, sudden pain or medical complication. More than just a metaphor, these services play a central role in acute medicine.

The multiplicity of cases
Emergency is a place of impressive clinical diversity. In the space of an hour, a nurse may be faced with a child with a fracture, an adult who has collapsed, or an elderly person with heart failure. This diversity demands adaptability, a broad knowledge base and the ability to prioritise quickly.

The art of triage
As soon as a patient arrives, the initial assessment, or triage, is essential. Triage nurses are trained to quickly assess the severity of symptoms, identify cases requiring immediate intervention and direct patients to the appropriate care. This process ensures that those in immediate danger receive attention first, even when the department is overloaded.

Care coordination
Emergency departments are not isolated. They constantly interact with other departments - radiology, laboratory, surgery and so on. The nurse often plays the role of coordinator, ensuring that the necessary tests are carried out quickly and that the appropriate specialists are consulted in good time.

Managing pressure

Emergency situations are inherently stressful. Nurses and doctors often have to make vital decisions in a matter of minutes, while managing their own emotions and those of patients and families. This pressure requires solid training, emotional resilience and constant team support.

Communication in chaos

In the midst of turmoil, clear and concise communication is essential. Whether it's informing a doctor of a change in condition, reassuring an anxious patient or coordinating with another team, the ability to convey accurate information can mean the difference between life and death.

Ethical and human challenges

Emergency situations often raise complex ethical questions: when should resuscitation be stopped? How should refusal of treatment be managed? Faced with these dilemmas, the team must come together, draw on solid ethical principles and, above all, put the patient at the centre of all decisions.

Emergency departments embody the quintessence of acute medicine. They are the place where medical theory meets the rawest reality, where clinical competence is continually put to the test and where the humanity of every healthcare professional is called upon at every moment. In this constant dance between science, ethics and emotion, the emergency department remains an essential pillar of the healthcare system, tirelessly looking after those who need it most.

The intensive care unit :
at the heart of gravity

If there's one place in a hospital where the fragility of life is felt at every moment, it's the intensive care unit (ICU).

Every machine that beeps, every monitor that displays curves, every carer who works around a bed, bears witness to the constant struggle between life and death. At the heart of acute medicine, the ICU is a sanctuary for the most critical cases.

Patients in critical condition
Patients admitted to the ICU suffer from failure of one or more vital organs. Whether suffering from respiratory failure requiring mechanical ventilation, septic shock or severe trauma, these patients require constant monitoring and intervention.

A highly technological environment
The ICU is a concentrate of advanced medical technology. Respirators, heart monitors, infusion pumps, dialysis machines - every piece of equipment plays a crucial role. But these machines are only tools. It is the skill, vigilance and expertise of the nurses and doctors who transform this technology into truly life-saving care.

Multidisciplinary collaboration
The ICU brings together a highly specialised team. As well as nurses and intensive care doctors, there are physiotherapists, nutritionists, pharmacologists and many others. This collaboration is essential for managing the complexity of cases and ensuring holistic patient care.

Decision-making in a hurry
In this environment, where every second counts, decision-making must be rapid, informed and evidence-based. This requires not only an in-depth knowledge of medicine, but also effective communication within the team and with patients' relatives.

Emotional and ethical issues
The ICU is also the scene of intensely emotional moments. Families experience anguish, hope and grief. Decisions to prolong treatment, limit care or donate organs are commonplace and require a rigorous ethical approach that is imbued with humanity.

The importance of psychological support
The emotional burden of the ICU does not only affect patients and their families. Healthcare professionals, faced with extreme situations on a daily basis, may experience stress, fatigue or even symptoms of post-traumatic distress. Psychological support, supervision and stress management training are therefore essential.

The intensive care unit is much more than just a hospital ward, it's a microcosm where science, the art of care and humanity intertwine. In this small space, every gesture counts, every decision carries weight, every moment shared is precious. And while the ICU bears witness to the extreme seriousness of certain medical conditions, it also powerfully illustrates the determination, commitment and unfailing compassion of those who work there.

Discharge rooms and observation rooms

When you think of a hospital emergency department, the images that often spring to mind are those of the wards and observation rooms. These areas, although distinct, are inseparable from the acute care process and represent key stages in the patient's journey.

Discharge rooms: life-saving intervention
Discharge wards are where patients in critical situations are cared for, requiring immediate interventions to stabilise their condition.
- **Equipment and preparation**: These rooms are equipped to deal with any emergency - from cardiopulmonary resuscitation to the treatment of serious trauma. They must be ready to receive a patient at any time.
- **The team in action**: Working in the out-patient department requires close collaboration between

doctors, nurses, care assistants and technicians. Each member of the team knows his or her role and what needs to be done, whether it's administering medication, preparing equipment or communicating with other departments.

- **Rapid decision-making**: When faced with a patient in distress, every second counts. Professionals need to assess the situation quickly, decide on the best course of action and carry it out without hesitation.

Observation rooms: close monitoring

After an initial operation, patients are often referred to observation rooms. These areas are designed to monitor patients' condition over a longer period, generally from a few hours to a day.

- **The importance of monitoring**: Even after stabilisation, patients may experience complications or changes in their condition. Observation rooms provide constant monitoring, ensuring rapid intervention if necessary.
- **Ongoing assessment**: During their stay in the observation room, patients are regularly assessed. Examinations, analyses and consultations with specialists help to refine the diagnosis and adjust treatment.
- **Preparing for what comes next**: The observation room is also where decisions are made about what happens next for the patient. Depending on their condition, they may be admitted to hospital, referred to another department or sent home with specific recommendations.

The discharge and observation rooms symbolise the two poles of the emergency continuum: immediate intervention in the event of a crisis and close monitoring pending complete stabilisation. These two environments, although different in function, share a common objective: to ensure the best possible care for each patient, at every stage of their stay in the emergency department. In these environments, medical expertise mingles with benevolence, efficiency with compassion, offering a response adapted to the complexity and urgency of the situations encountered.

Chapter 3.
CORE COMPETENCIES
IN ACUTE MEDICINE

Quick and efficient assessment

• The art of sorting

Triage, derived from the French word "trier", is a fundamental element of the medical world, particularly in the emergency context. It is a process by which healthcare professionals assess the urgency and severity of patients' conditions in order to determine the priority of care. Although it may seem like simple ranking, triage is a delicate art that combines medical knowledge, clinical intuition and compassion.

The need for triage

In a context where resources, whether in terms of time, staff or equipment, are limited, it is crucial to quickly identify those who need immediate intervention. This ensures that patients who are most at risk see a doctor first, regardless of the order in which they arrive.

The main assessment criteria

Triage is not based on a single sign or symptom. Instead, the triage nurse assesses a combination of factors:

- **Main symptoms**: What are the signs and symptoms presented? Chest pain, for example, will often be treated with higher priority than a sprained ankle.
- **Vital signs**: Parameters such as heart rate, blood pressure, respiratory rate and temperature may indicate medical distress.
- **General appearance**: Sometimes, simply observing the patient can provide clues. A pale, sweaty or obviously distressed patient is a warning sign.

Triage levels

Most triage systems classify patients into several categories, ranging from those requiring immediate intervention to those who can wait longer. These levels ensure that resources are allocated efficiently.

The importance of communication

An essential aspect of triage is the ability to communicate effectively with patients to obtain a clear medical history in a limited time. In addition, it is crucial to explain to patients and their families why some have to wait longer than others, in order to minimise anxiety and frustration.

Training and updating skills

The medical world is constantly evolving, and triage protocols are no exception. Triage nurses need regular training and to be up to date with the latest recommendations and research to ensure accurate and effective triage.

The emotional challenges of triage

Triaging patients, some with minor complaints, others in life-threatening situations, can be emotionally draining. Professionals not only have to manage their own emotions, but also those of patients and families, who are often anxious or frightened.

The art of triage is a delicate dance between urgency, gravity, resourcefulness and compassion. It is the crucial first step in a life-saving care pathway. By understanding the subtleties and challenges of triage, we can better appreciate the importance of this process and the dedication of those who practice it.

• Initial assessment techniques

The initial assessment of a patient is one of the most crucial stages in the medical management process, particularly in acute medicine. It provides the healthcare professional with a first impression that will guide further investigations and interventions. This assessment is a combination of observations, targeted questions and physical examinations, all carried out in a short space of time to maximise the effectiveness of the treatment.

1. Systematic approach :
An assessment process must be methodical to ensure that no crucial element is omitted.

- **A - Airways**: Make sure the patient's airways are clear.
- **B - Breathing**: Assess the quality, frequency and regularity of breathing.
- **C - Circulation**: Check pulse, skin colour, and look for signs of shock.
- **D - Neurological deficit**: Assess level of consciousness, pupil size and reactivity, and motor and sensory function.
- **E - Exposure/Environmental examination**: Exposing the patient to look for any hidden injuries, while preserving his or her privacy and protecting him or her from external elements.

2. Anamnesis using the SAMPLE technique :
- **S (Symptoms)**: How the patient feels.
- **A (Allergies)** : Any known allergy.
- **M (Medication)**: The medicines the patient is currently taking.
- **P (Medical history)** : Relevant medical history.
- **L (Last Meal)**: Last meal, useful in the event of anaesthesia or surgery.
- **E (Events)** : Events surrounding the current situation.

3. Targeted physical examination :
Depending on the patient's complaints and symptoms, a focused physical examination is carried out. If a patient complains of chest pain, for example, cardiac and pulmonary auscultation would be a priority.

4. Assessment of vital signs :
- **Heart rate**: Indicates the speed at which the heart beats.
- **Respiratory frequency**: Number of breaths per minute.
- **Arterial pressure**: Measure of the force of blood against the walls of the arteries.
- **Temperature**: Potential indication of infection or other conditions.
- **Oxygen saturation:** Measurement of the amount of oxygen in the blood.

5. Use of diagnostic equipment :
Devices such as the electrocardiogram (ECG), oxygen saturation monitor and others can be used to provide a more comprehensive initial assessment.

6. Active listening and observation :
In addition to physical examinations and questioning, careful observation of the patient's behaviour, appearance and interactions can provide valuable clues to their condition.

Initial assessment is a dynamic process that requires extensive training, practice, clinical intuition and the ability to act quickly on the information gathered. It is this first impression that will often guide subsequent care, making this one of the most vital stages in the treatment of patients in acute medicine.

Emergency techniques : from resuscitation to intubation

Emergency situations in acute medicine require rapid, decisive action based on precise technical skills to save lives. In this world, certain interventions, such as cardiopulmonary resuscitation (CPR) and intubation, are among the most critical. They require not only specialist training, but also the ability to remain calm under pressure.

1. Cardiopulmonary resuscitation (CPR)
- **Objective**: To restore blood circulation and oxygenation when the heart stops beating.
  - Technical details :
    - **Positioning**: Lay the patient down on a hard surface and position yourself next to them.
    - **Compression**: With your hands on top of each other, apply firm, rapid pressure to the sternum, allowing the heart to fill between each compression.
    - **Ventilation**: After 30 compressions, give two breaths (if trained to do so), either by mouth-to-mouth or using a barrier mask.

2. Defibrillation
- **Objective**: To treat ventricular fibrillation or pulseless ventricular tachycardia by delivering an electric shock to the heart.
  - Technical details :
    - **Preparation**: Ensure that the patient is disconnected from any conductive devices. Place the electrodes/pads on the chest according to the manufacturer's instructions.
    - **Defibrillation**: Select the appropriate energy, tell everyone to move away, then deliver the shock.

3. Airway management
- **Objective: To** ensure a clear airway for effective ventilation.
  - Technical details :
    - **Positioning**: Use subluxation of the head and elevation of the chin or mandible to open the airway.

- **Aspiration**: If secretions or vomit are obstructing the airways, use an aspirator to remove them.

4. Intubation
  - **Objective**: To establish a protected airway and ensure adequate ventilation, particularly in situations where spontaneous ventilation is compromised.
    - Technical details :
    - **Preparation**: Gather together all the necessary materials, including the laryngoscope, endotracheal tube, stethoscope and tube attachment.
    - **Positioning**: Place the patient in the "sniffing" position (cervical extension and atlanto-occipital flexion).
    - **Visualisation**: Insert the blade of the laryngoscope into the mouth, move the tongue and visualise the vocal cords.
    - **Tube insertion**: Slide the endotracheal tube through the vocal cords while visualising.
    - **Confirmation**: Confirm the position using methods such as auscultation, condensation visualisation or a capnograph.

Each of these techniques requires not only technical mastery, but also the ability to collaborate effectively with the entire medical team. In the tumultuous environment of the emergency room, success often depends on a combination of individual skills and impeccable team coordination. These interventions are the very essence of emergency medicine, where every second counts and lives are often at stake.

Communication in crisis situations

• Working with the medical team

In the fast-paced and complex world of acute medicine, collaboration within the medical team is essential to ensure safe and effective patient care. This chapter explores the dynamics of collaboration between the nurse and the various members of the medical team, and how this synergy promotes better care.

1. Understanding the role of each member
   - **The doctor**: a clinical leader, he or she makes diagnoses, prescribes treatments and monitors patients' progress.
   - **The nurse**: Plays a pivotal role in coordinating care, administering medication, monitoring patients and providing education.
   - **The laboratory technician**: Analyses samples to guide diagnosis and monitoring.
   - **The radiologist**: Interprets medical images, providing crucial information for diagnosis.
   - **Paramedical professionals**: Physiotherapists, occupational therapists, nutritionists, etc., all bring their specialist skills to bear on patient care.
   - **Administrative staff**: manage the logistical and organisational aspects, ensuring that the unit runs smoothly.
2. Effective communication
   - **Active listening**: Lending an attentive ear to the concerns and suggestions of each member.
   - **Feedback**: Ensure a communication loop, particularly when passing on instructions.
   - **Use of standardised tools**: Shared checklists, warning systems and protocols ensure mutual understanding.

3. Collaborative decision-making
- **Multidisciplinary discussion**: Regular meetings to discuss complex cases and establish a coherent care plan.
- **Making the most of each member's skills**: Recognising and making the most of individual expertise to improve care.

4. Conflict management
- **Proactive resolution**: Tackling problems as soon as they arise, before they get worse.
- **Mediation**: If necessary, bring in a third party to facilitate resolution.
- **Interpersonal skills training**: Regular sessions to strengthen communication and mutual understanding.

5. Ongoing training and education
- **Joint training**: Sessions where different professions learn together to improve collaboration.
- **Role-playing**: Understanding the responsibilities of others, reinforcing empathy and cooperation.

Collaboration within the medical team is the beating heart of acute medicine. It transcends simple professional interactions to create an environment where the patient is at the centre of a constellation of experts, each bringing their own unique light to illuminate the path to recovery. The nurse, as the central link in this team, plays a crucial role in facilitating this collaboration.

• Communicating with patients and their families

Communication is at the heart of nursing care. In the stressful context of acute medicine, knowing how to establish a dialogue with patients and their relatives is not only essential for providing quality care, but also for building a relationship of trust. This chapter explores the nuances of this communication, techniques for facilitating it, and the importance of compassion and empathy.

1. Making initial contact
   - **Calm approach**: A gentle entrance to the room, a soothing tone of voice and an open posture help to reassure the patient.
   - **Clear presentation**: Always introduce yourself and explain your role.
   - **Active listening**: Letting the patient express his or her concerns without interruption.
2. Effective communication techniques
   - **Appropriate language**: Avoid medical jargon and ensure that the patient and those close to them understand the information.
   - **Open questioning**: Encourage the patient to speak freely by asking open questions.
   - **Reformulation**: Repeating what the patient has said to confirm mutual understanding.
3. Managing emotions
   - **Recognising signs of distress**: Crying, agitation, silence or anger require a sensitive approach.
   - **Bringing comfort**: A simple human touch, like a hand on the shoulder, can bring great comfort.
   - **Space for grief**: In the most difficult situations, give loved ones the space and time they need to express their emotions.
4. Inform without overloading
   - **Prioritising information**: Determining what the patient and family absolutely need to know, and what can be discussed later.
   - **Written documents**: Providing brochures or information sheets can help consolidate understanding.

5. Communicating with family and friends
- **Confidentiality**: Always ask the patient's permission before sharing medical information with family and friends.
- **Involvement in care**: Encourage relatives to ask questions and take part in care, wherever possible.

6. Managing difficult situations
- **Bad news**: Adopt a gentle, empathetic approach, ensure a private environment and provide emotional support.
- **Conflicts**: Listen to concerns, remain calm and call in a mediator if necessary.

7. Follow-up
- **Recheck**: Return regularly to ensure that the patient and those close to them understand and are comfortable with the care plan.
- **Additional resources**: Provide contacts or referrals for additional support, such as support groups or counselling services.

Communicating with patients and their families involves much more than simply passing on information. It is a delicate art that requires empathy, patience and compassion. In the tumult of acute medicine, this communication humanises care, reminding us at every moment that behind every diagnosis lies a person with hopes, fears and dreams.

Chapter 4.
Common pathologies and nursing care

Cardiovascular disorders

• Myocardial infarction

Myocardial infarction, commonly known as heart attack, is a medical emergency characterised by the death of part of the heart muscle due to a lack of oxygen supply. It is one of the leading causes of death worldwide. Understanding myocardial infarction, its causes, symptoms and management is essential for all healthcare professionals working in acute medicine.

1. Anatomy and physiology of the heart
   - **The heart muscle (myocardium)**: its structure, function and importance in blood circulation.
   - **Coronary arteries**: The vessels responsible for supplying oxygen to the heart.
2. Causes and mechanisms of infarction
   - **Atherosclerosis**: The build-up of cholesterol plaques in the arteries, reducing blood flow.
   - **Coronary thrombosis**: the formation of a clot that blocks a coronary artery, depriving part of the heart of oxygen.
   - **Risk factors**: Smoking, hypertension, diabetes, obesity, family history, etc.
3. Symptoms of heart attack
   - **Chest pain**: Often described as pressure, crushing or pain radiating to the arm, jaw or back.
   - Shortness of breath
   - Sweating, nausea or dizziness
   - **Atypical symptoms**: Especially in women, the elderly or diabetics.

4. Diagnosis of infarction
- **Electrocardiogram (ECG)**: Measures the electrical activity of the heart, revealing areas of damage.
- **Blood tests**: Measure the cardiac enzymes released during damage to the myocardium.
- **Coronary angiography:** An imaging technique that visualises the coronary arteries.

5. Emergency care
- **Stabilising the patient**: monitoring vital signs, administering oxygen and pain medication.
- **Reperfusion**: Rapid restoration of blood flow, either by thrombolysis (clot-dissolving drugs) or percutaneous coronary intervention (angioplasty).
- **Medication**: Beta-blockers, anticoagulants, statins and others to treat and prevent other cardiac events.

6. Recovery and rehabilitation
- **Post-infarction care**: Monitoring in the intensive care unit, assessment of cardiac function, and long-term treatment planning.
- **Cardiac rehabilitation**: Supervised programmes combining exercise, education and support to help patients return to a normal life and prevent another heart attack.
- **Lifestyle changes**: Stop smoking, healthy diet, regular exercise and stress management.

7. Preventing heart attacks
- **Controlling risk factors**: high blood pressure, cholesterol, diabetes.
- **Preventive medication**: Aspirin, statins, antihypertensives.
- **Patient education**: Recognising the warning signs and when to seek help.

A myocardial infarction is a serious medical event that requires rapid and competent intervention. With appropriate treatment, many patients can recover and live a full and active life. However, prevention remains the key to reducing the risk of heart attack and its potentially fatal complications.

• Acute heart failure

Heart failure is a condition in which the heart is unable to pump blood adequately to meet the body's needs. Acute heart failure (AHF) represents a rapid deterioration or first manifestation of heart failure, often requiring urgent medical attention.

1. Understanding the disease
   * **Cardiac physiology**: How the heart functions normally to ensure blood circulation.
   * **Types of failure**: Left, right or global heart failure.
2. Causes of acute heart failure
   * Coronary heart disease
   * Uncontrolled hypertension
   * Valvulopathy
   * Cardiomyopathies
   * Heart rhythm disorders
   * **Other**: infections, drug toxicities, etc.
3. Symptoms and clinical signs
   * Shortness of breath
   * Pulmonary oedema
   * Extreme fatigue
   * Swelling of the legs, ankles and feet
   * Persistent or wheezing cough
   * Rapid weight gain
4. Diagnosis
   * **Listen for heart sounds**: identify murmurs and crackles in the lungs.
   * **Echocardiography**: Direct visualisation of heart function.
   * **Chest X-ray**: Identification of pulmonary congestion.
   * **Blood tests**: Measurement of BNP (brain natriuretic peptide) levels, a marker of CIA.

5. Therapeutic management
- **Stabilisation**: administration of oxygen, semi-seated position.
  - Medicines :
  - **Diuretics**: To reduce excess fluid.
  - **Vasodilators**: To dilate blood vessels.
  - **Inotropes** : To improve cardiac contractility.
- **Ventilatory assistance**: In serious cases where the patient cannot obtain sufficient oxygen.
- **Advanced treatments**: ventricular assist devices, heart transplantation.
6. Education and follow-up
- **Self-monitoring**: Teaching patients to recognise the precursor symptoms of an exacerbation.
- **Lifestyle changes**: low-salt diet, weight management, medication monitoring.
- **Action plan**: When and how to seek medical help.
7. Prevention
- **Management of underlying diseases**: Blood pressure control, treatment of coronary heart disease.
- **Vaccinations**: Prevent respiratory infections, which can aggravate CIA.
- **Avoiding triggers**: Excessive consumption of fluids or salt, certain non-prescribed medications.

Acute heart failure is a serious condition requiring rapid medical management. Early intervention, combined with appropriate patient education, can significantly improve prognosis and quality of life.

Respiratory problems

• Severe acute asthma
Asthma is a chronic inflammatory disease of the airways characterised by recurrent episodes of coughing,

wheezing, breathlessness and chest tightness. Severe acute asthma, often referred to as an "asthma attack", represents an intense exacerbation of these symptoms, potentially life-threatening and requiring immediate medical intervention.

1. Understanding asthma
   - **Pulmonary anatomy**: Function and structure of the airways.
   - **Pathophysiology of asthma**: Inflammation, bronchoconstriction and mucus hypersecretion.
2. Triggering factors
   - **Allergens**: Pollen, dust mites, mould, animal hair.
   - **Irritants**: Tobacco smoke, air pollution, perfumes.
   - Respiratory infections: colds, flu.
   - Emotional factors: Stress, anxiety.
   - **Other**: Medication, exercise without a warm-up, weather conditions.
3. Symptoms and signs of severe acute asthma
   - Rapid, shallow breathing
   - Chest wheezing audible at a distance
   - Interspersed speech
   - Visible anxiety or panic
   - Use of accessory muscles for breathing
   - Cyanosis (bluish discolouration of the skin)
4. Diagnosis
   - **Clinical assessment**: Observing and listening to the airways.
   - **Spirometry**: Measurement of respiratory volumes and flows (often limited in crisis situations).
   - **Oxygen saturation**: Using a pulse oximeter.
5. Therapeutic management
   - **Rapid-acting bronchodilators**: Salbutamol or terbutaline, generally administered by inhaler or nebuliser.
   - **Systemic steroids**: such as prednisolone to reduce inflammation.

- **Oxygen**: For patients in respiratory distress or with low oxygen saturation.
- **Close monitoring**: Regular assessment of vital signs, respiratory function and oxygen saturation.
- **Hospitalisation**: In cases where the seizure does not respond quickly to treatment or is particularly severe.

6. Education and prevention
- **Asthma action plan: a** written, personalised tool to help patients recognise and manage early exacerbations.
- **Trigger management**: Identifying and minimising exposure to personal triggers.
- **Emergency inhalers**: Always have a fast-acting bronchodilator to hand.
- **Inhalation techniques**: Ensure that patients use their inhalation devices correctly.

7. Regular monitoring
- **Follow-up consultations**: Regular assessment of lung function, severity of symptoms and adjustment of medication.
- **Vaccinations**: against influenza and pneumonia to reduce the risk of exacerbations.

A severe acute asthma attack is a medical emergency requiring rapid intervention. Good patient education, combined with a personalised management plan, can help prevent many exacerbations and ensure prompt care when necessary.

• Pulmonary embolism

Pulmonary embolism (PE) is a potentially fatal condition caused by a blood clot that migrates to the lungs, usually obstructing one or more pulmonary arteries. This compromises blood flow to the lungs and can affect the body's ability to oxygenate the blood.

1. Understanding pulmonary embolism
   - **Lung physiology**: How the lungs receive blood for oxygenation.
   - **Thrombosis and embolism**: Formation and migration of clots.
2. Causes and risk factors
   - **Deep vein thrombosis (DVT)**: formation of a clot in the deep veins, usually in the legs, which can break loose and migrate to the lungs.
   - **Prolonged immobilisation**: Hospitalisation, long-haul travel.
   - **Surgery**: Particularly orthopaedic or abdomino-pelvic surgery.
   - Cancer.
   - Pregnancy and the post-partum period.
   - **Hormonal treatments**: oral contraceptives, hormone replacement therapy.
   - Genetic conditions: Thrombophilias.
3. Symptoms and clinical signs
   - Sudden shortness of breath.
   - **Chest pain**: aggravated by deep breathing.
   - **Cough**: Sometimes with blood.
   - Cyanosis.
   - Tachycardia.
   - Syncope or dizziness.
4. Diagnosis
   - **Pulmonary angiography**: Gold standard, but rarely used.
   - Lung scintigraphy.
   - Doppler ultrasound of the lower limbs: to look for associated DVT.
   - Lung computed tomography (CT) with injection: Increasingly common.
   - **Blood tests**: D-dimer to exclude the diagnosis.
5. Therapeutic management
   - **Anticoagulation:** Low molecular weight heparin, warfarin or direct oral anticoagulants.

- **Thrombolysis: In cases of** massive PE or haemodynamic instability.
- **Vena filter**: For patients with a contraindication to anticoagulation.
- **Surgical embolectomy**: Rarely used, except in extreme cases.

6. Prevention
- **Anticoagulant prophylaxis** : For patients at risk during hospitalisation or after certain surgical procedures.
- **Compression stockings**: Reduce the risk of DVT.
- **Early mobilisation**: After surgery or during prolonged hospitalisation.

7. Education and follow-up
- **Recognising symptoms**: the importance of prompt treatment.
- **Anticoagulants**: Education on signs of bleeding, drug interactions and regular monitoring.
- **Modifiable risk factors**: Encourage people to stop smoking, lose weight if necessary and reduce hormonal risk factors.

Pulmonary embolism is a medical emergency requiring rapid intervention and appropriate management. Recognition of symptoms, prevention in patients at risk and patient education on anticoagulants are essential to reduce the morbidity and mortality associated with this condition.

Sepsis and septic shock

Sepsis is an extreme bodily response to infection that can lead to tissue damage, organ failure and death. Septic shock is a complication of sepsis characterised by profound and persistent arterial hypotension despite adequate vascular filling, leading to insufficient perfusion of the organs.

1. Definition and understanding
   - **Sepsis:** Systemic inflammatory response to infection.
   - **Septic shock**: sepsis with tissue hypoperfusion despite adequate volume resuscitation.
2. Causes and risk factors
   - **Bacterial infections**: More frequent, including pneumonia, urinary tract infections and peritonitis.
   - Viral, fungal or parasitic infections: Less common, but possible.
   - **Immunosuppression**: Cancer, chemotherapy, steroids, HIV.
   - Advanced age.
   - **Chronic conditions**: diabetes, kidney or heart failure.
   - **Medical interventions**: catheters, surgery, mechanical ventilation.
3. Symptoms and clinical signs
   - Fever or hypothermia.
   - Tachycardia.
   - **Tachypnoea** or hyperventilation.
   - Altered mental state: Confusion, drowsiness.
   - **Arterial hypotension** (particularly in septic shock).
   - **Oliguria**: reduced urine output.
4. Diagnosis
   - **Blood tests**: Increase in leucocytes, rise in lactates, coagulation disturbances.
   - **Blood cultures**: Identify the infectious agent.
   - **Imaging**: Chest X-ray, CT scan, ultrasound to locate the source of infection.
   - **Samples**: Urine, CSF, pleural or peritoneal fluid for culture.
5. Therapeutic management
   - **Empirical antibiotic therapy**: Rapid administration of broad-spectrum antibiotics.
   - **Volume resuscitation**: crystalloids or even colloids.

- **Haemodynamic support**: Vasopressors such as norepinephrine in cases of septic shock.
- **Organ support if necessary**: mechanical ventilation, dialysis.
- **Source control**: Drainage, surgery or removal of a medical device if this is the source of the infection.

6. Complications
- **Multiple organ dysfunction**: Multiple organ damage due to inflammation and hypoperfusion.
- **Coagulopathy**: Coagulation disorders that may lead to bleeding or thrombosis.
- Acute renal failure.

7. Prevention and education
- **Hygiene**: hand washing, asepsis techniques.
- **Vaccinations**: Prevention of infections that can lead to sepsis.
- **Recognising early signs**: the importance of rapid medical intervention in the event of suspicion.
- **Post-sepsis follow-up**: Monitoring of potential after-effects and psychological support.

Sepsis and septic shock are major medical emergencies. Prompt recognition and appropriate, intensive treatment are essential to reduce the mortality and sequelae associated with these conditions. Targeted education of healthcare professionals and the general public is essential to improve outcomes.

Trauma and injuries

Trauma and injuries are bodily injuries resulting from external physical forces. They can range from a simple bruise to life-threatening injuries. The role of the nurse is crucial in assessing, stabilising and treating these patients, while working closely with the medical team.

1. Classification of trauma
   - **Closed trauma**: No break in the skin (e.g. contusion, non-open fracture).
   - **Open trauma**: Skin breakage (e.g. wounds, open fractures).
   - **Penetrating trauma**: Injuries caused by sharp objects or projectiles (e.g. bullet wounds, knife wounds).
2. Mechanisms of injury
   - Falls.
   - **Road accidents**: pedestrians, cyclists, motorists.
   - Crushing.
   - Sharp or puncture wounds.
   - **Burns**: Thermal, chemical, electrical.
   - **Violence**: Domestic, assault, fighting.
3. Initial assessment
   - **ABCDE approach**: Airways (A), Breathing (B), Circulation (C), Neurological deficit (D), Exposure/ Environment (E).
   - **Triage**: Assess severity and prioritise care.
   - **Full physical examination**: looking for hidden lesions.

4. Therapeutic management
   - **Stabilisation**: Immobilisation, oxygenation, venous access.
   - **Resuscitation**: In the event of cardiopulmonary arrest.
   - Pain management: Analgesia.
   - **Surgery**: To treat fractures, internal haemorrhage or other injuries.
5. Monitoring complications
   - **Haemorrhage**: External and internal.
   - **Organ dysfunction**: Respiratory failure, renal failure.
   - **Infections**: On open wound sites.
   - **Neurological complications**: head injuries, spinal cord injuries.

6. Psychological support
- **Post-traumatic stress management**: listening, support, referral to specialists.
- Communicating with patients and their families: providing information, reassurance and support.

7. Injury prevention
- **Public education**: Road safety campaigns, prevention of falls among the elderly.
- **Protective equipment**: Helmets, seatbelts, reflective waistcoats.

8. Re-education and rehabilitation
- **Physiotherapy**: To restore mobility after fractures or operations.
- **Occupational therapy**: Helping people regain their independence in everyday activities.
- **Medical follow-up**: To check healing and prevent after-effects.

Trauma and injury are common in emergency medicine. Nurses play a pivotal role in the care of these patients, from their arrival in the emergency department to their referral to a suitable specialty or discharge. Speed, precision and coordination with the medical team are essential to ensure the best possible care.

Chapter 5.
THE PSYCHOLOGICAL DIMENSION
ACUTE MEDICINE

Managing stress and burnout

Acute medicine is a demanding and stressful field, where nurses are frequently confronted with life-and-death situations. This constant pressure, coupled with long working hours and interaction with patients and families who are often anxious or distressed, can lead to intense stress and burnout. It is essential for nurses to understand, recognise and manage these challenges to ensure optimal patient care and to safeguard their own well-being.

1. Understanding stress and burnout
   - **Definitions**: Differentiation between daily stress, chronic stress and burnout.
   - **Causes in the medical context**: Pressure, emergencies, emotional management, patient-caregiver interaction.
2. Recognising signs and symptoms
   - **Physical**: Fatigue, sleep disorders, headaches, gastrointestinal problems.
   - **Emotional**: Irritability, feelings of inadequacy, detachment, anxiety.
   - **Behavioural**: Procrastination, task avoidance, neglect of responsibilities.
3. Impact on patient care
   - **Risk of medical errors**: hasty decisions, oversights, negligence.
   - **Patient-caregiver interactions**: Less empathy, impaired communication, patient dissatisfaction.

4. Stress management strategies
- **Relaxation techniques**: deep breathing, meditation, yoga.
- **Time management**: planning, delegation, breaks.
- **Professional limits**: Recognising your limits, knowing how to say no, taking days off.

5. Preventing burnout
- **Supervision and mentoring**: Support from experienced colleagues.
- **Ongoing training**: stress management techniques, communication, leadership.
- **Work-life balance**: Make sure you have time for yourself, your family and your hobbies.

6. Importance of support
- **Multidisciplinary teams**: working together, sharing responsibilities.
- **Therapy and counselling**: Having a space to discuss and process your emotions.
- **Support groups**: Exchanging ideas with colleagues facing the same challenges.

7. Resources available
- **Institutional programmes**: Well-being programmes, psychological consultations.
- **Professional organisations**: nursing associations, trade unions.
- **Literature and training**: Books, seminars and webinars on stress management and preventing burnout.

8. Recognition and action
- **Acknowledge reality**: Acknowledge that no one is immune to stress or exhaustion.
- **Asking for help**: Turn to colleagues, management or a professional.

Nurses are an essential link in the care chain. To ensure optimal care, it is crucial that they are in good mental and physical health. Recognising and managing stress and burnout is a fundamental step in ensuring the quality of care and well-being of nurses.

Supporting patients in critical moments

In acute medicine, nurses are often the first point of contact for patients and their families at difficult times, whether it's a serious diagnosis, resuscitation or an uncertain prognosis. In these situations, the nurse's ability to offer empathetic and competent support is essential for the patient's well-being and to establish a relationship of trust.

1. Recognising the emotional impact
   - **Recognising the patient's vulnerability**: emotional reactions, fears and anxieties.
   - **Understanding the role of relatives**: their feelings of powerlessness, their need for information and support.
2. Empathetic communication
   - **Active listening**: Giving patients the space and time to express their feelings.
   - **Avoid medical jargon**: express yourself clearly and simply.
   - **Validating the patient's emotions**: Recognising and accepting their feelings without judgement.
3. Provide clear and precise information
   - **Remain honest**: Do not hide or minimise the seriousness of a situation.
   - **Offer explanations**: Help patients understand their medical situation.
   - **Answering questions**: Take the time to clarify any doubts or concerns.
4. A reassuring physical presence
   - **Therapeutic touch**: A simple hand on the shoulder can bring comfort.

- **Posture**: Get down to the patient's level and maintain eye contact.

5. Involving the patient in decision-making
   - **Offering choices**: Even in critical situations, patients can have preferences.
   - **Respecting patients' autonomy**: recognising their right to accept or refuse certain types of care.

6. Supporting relatives
   - **Providing a space to talk**: Relatives also need to express their emotions.
   - **Providing resources**: Informing people about available support services, such as social workers or psychologists.

7. Working with the care team
   - **Exchanging with doctors**: Having up-to-date information on the patient's condition.
   - **Helping colleagues**: sharing your feelings and approach strategies.

8. Protecting yourself emotionally
   - **Recognise your own limitations**: accept that you cannot always "cure" a patient's ill-being.
   - **Find spaces to decompress**: take breaks, talk to colleagues, use personal support resources.

9. Post-crisis reflections
   - **Debriefings with the team**: Analysing what went well and areas for improvement.
   - **Feedback from patients and relatives: to** enable them to express their feelings about the care provided.

10. Further training
   - Developing communication skills: training, simulations, role-plays.
   - **Familiarising yourself with psychological support tools**: learning to recognise and manage symptoms of distress.

Supporting a patient at a critical time is one of the noblest, but also most demanding tasks for a nurse. It requires a combination of professional skill, emotional understanding and personal resilience. It's at times like these that the human side of nursing really comes into its own.

The importance of debriefing after major events

At the heart of acute medical services, nurses are regularly exposed to stressful, unexpected and sometimes traumatic situations. Whether following a complex resuscitation, an unexpected event or a death, post-event debriefing is an essential tool. Post-event debriefing is not just a stress management technique, but a comprehensive approach that promotes resilience, learning and continuous improvement in the quality of care.

1. Defining debriefing
   - **What is a debrief?** A structured post-event discussion.
   - **The main objectives are to** understand, learn and support.
2. Psychological benefits
   - **Expressing and processing emotions**: A safe space to talk about your feelings.
   - **Reducing the risk of post-traumatic stress disorder**: Recognising and tackling early symptoms.
   - **Enhancing collective support**: Strengthening the sense of belonging and solidarity within the team.
3. Encouraging learning
   - **Identify successes**: Recognise what has worked well.

- **Analyse areas for improvement**: Without passing judgement, consider how you can do things better in the future.
- **Action plan for the future**: Implement concrete solutions to avoid repeating mistakes.

4. Improving communication within the team

- **Encouraging interdisciplinary exchange**: bringing together different perspectives for a global understanding.
- **Strengthening team cohesion**: Valuing collective work and the importance of each member.
- **Developing a feedback culture**: Encouraging open and constructive communication.

5. Optimising the quality of care

- **Identify system flaws**: Identify structural or organisational problems.
- **Implementing changes**: Adjust protocols or practices based on feedback.
- **Monitor and evaluate improvements**: Measure the impact of changes made.

6. Structuring the debriefing

- **When should it be carried out?** Ideally soon after the event, but taking into account the immediate needs of the department.
- **Who should take part?** Any member of the team involved, and possibly an external facilitator.
- **How should it be conducted?** With an open mind, without judgement, following a framework or guide.

7. Debriefing and ethics

- **Confidentiality**: Ensuring that discussions remain within the team.
- **Non-judgement** : Adopting a stance of listening and mutual understanding.
- **Respect for each participant**: Everyone should feel free to express themselves without fear of repercussions.

8. Training in debriefing
- **Learn facilitation techniques**: how to guide a constructive discussion.
- **Recognise signs of distress**: Refer to professional support if necessary.
- **Integrate debriefing into the team culture**: make it a regular practice, not just after major events.

Concluding a major event with a debriefing does not mean simply "turning the page", but rather building on the experience to strengthen the team, improve professional practice and ensure the best possible quality of care for future patients.

Chapter 6.
ETHICS AND LAW IN ACUTE MEDICINE

Consent and capacity

In the medical world, respect for patient autonomy is a fundamental principle. Informed consent and the ability to give that consent are at the heart of this principle. However, in acute medicine, where decisions often need to be made quickly and patients may be in altered states, navigating these areas can be complex. It is an area that requires both a deep understanding of the ethical and legal aspects, as well as the ability to communicate effectively.

1. Fundamental principles
   - **What is informed consent**: A voluntary decision based on full information.
   - **Understanding capacity**: The ability to understand and appreciate the consequences of one's decisions.
2. Assess capacity
   - **Criteria for assessing ability**: Understanding information, assessing the situation, reasoning and communicating a decision.
   - **Factors that can influence capacity**: Medication, mental illness, acute conditions such as delirium, etc.
   - **Interdisciplinary assessment**: collaboration with professionals such as psychiatrists or social workers.
3. Obtaining informed consent
   - **Provide comprehensive information**: nature of the intervention, benefits, risks, alternatives.
   - **Make sure the patient understands**: use clear language, check understanding, encourage questions.

- **Documenting consent**: Important for legal and ethical reasons.
4. Special situations
    - **Unconscious or seriously ill patients**: Use of advance directives or a legal representative.
    - **Minors and consent**: Capacity versus legal age of consent.
    - Emergency situations where consent cannot be obtained: life-saving interventions, legal framework.
5. Refusal of treatment
    - **Respecting autonomy**: Even if it goes against medical advice.
    - **Assess capacity**: Ensure refusal is based on intact capacity.
    - **Consequences and responsibilities**: Inform the patient, document carefully.
6. Advance directives and mandates
    - When they come into play: In the absence of capacity.
    - **Importance of updating**: Situations and wishes can change.
    - **Proactive discussion with patients**: Encourage patients to think about and document their wishes.
7. Ethical dilemmas
    - Conflicts between the medical team and the patient or family: negotiation, mediation.
    - Respect for autonomy versus benefit for the patient: When the patient's interest is at stake.
    - **Collegial decisions**: consulting peers, ethics committees.
8. Importance of communication
    - **Empathetic communication techniques**: active listening, validation of emotions.
    - **Managing disagreements**: patient-centred approach, seeking common ground.
    - **Include family and friends**: They can provide valuable information and support the decision-making process.

Respect for consent and capacity is essential to maintaining patient dignity and rights, even in emergency situations. Every nurse must be equipped to navigate these sometimes troubled waters with skill, compassion and clarity.

End-of-life care in an acute context

Providing end-of-life care in an acute setting can be one of the most complex and emotionally charged challenges a nurse can face. The rapid, interventionist approach typical of acute medicine often contrasts with the needs of a terminally ill patient, where comfort, dignity and emotional support may take precedence over curative interventions. This chapter explores the subtleties of providing this essential care in an acute setting.

1. Recognising the terminal phase
   - **Understanding the signs**: physiological changes, symptoms and indicator behaviours.
   - **Communication with the team**: working together to recognise and understand the disease trajectory.
   - **Respecting the patient's wishes**: advance directives, previous discussions and expressed wishes.
2. Redefining care objectives
   - **From curative to palliative**: transition from interventions aimed at curing to those aimed at relieving.
   - **The decision not to resuscitate (DNR)**: Understanding, respecting and communicating directives.
   - **Withdrawal of intensive interventions**: Deciding when and how to stop treatments such as ventilation or dialysis.

3. Symptom management
- **Pain**: assessment, medicinal and non-medicinal treatments.
- **Shortness of breath**: Relieve breathlessness without making the situation worse.
- **Agitation and delirium**: Recognising and managing these states to ensure maximum comfort.
- **Other common symptoms**: Nausea, constipation, xerostomia.

4. Emotional and spiritual support
- **Accompanying the patient**: Active listening, comforting presence.
- **Support for family and friends**: Helping with bereavement, providing a space for the expression of emotions.
- **Spiritual care services**: integration of chaplains or spiritual advisers into the care plan.

5. Communication
- **Delivering difficult news**: Techniques for sharing sensitive information.
- **Facilitating end-of-life discussions**: Exploring the patient's wishes and concerns.
- **Mediating disagreements**: negotiating and finding common ground between the medical team, the patient and the family.

6. Cultural and ethical aspects
- **Respecting cultural beliefs and practices**: Understanding and integrating diverse cultural perspectives.
- **Ethical decisions**: Navigating dilemmas such as artificial nutrition or hydration.

7. Self-care for the professional
- **Recognising emotional exhaustion**: Signs and symptoms of burnout.
- **Resilience strategies**: relaxation techniques, peer support, supervision.

- **Debriefing after a death**: Sharing, reflecting and learning from each experience.
8. Post-mortem
  - **Care of the body**: Respect, dignity and post-death procedures.
  - **Support for families after a death**: bereavement counselling, resources and guidance.

Caring for a terminally ill patient in an acute setting requires a unique combination of technical skill and compassion. It is essential to approach each situation with empathy, respect and openness, while providing the best possible care to ensure the comfort and dignity of the patient and their family.

Documentation and confidentiality

In the healthcare sector, accurate and complete documentation is crucial, not only to ensure continuity of quality care, but also to respect patients' legal and ethical rights. Confidentiality, meanwhile, lies at the heart of the relationship of trust between patient and healthcare team. Addressing these issues in an acute medical environment, where urgency and speed are often the order of the day, requires particular expertise.

1. Importance of documentation
  - **Continuity of care**: how accurate documentation promotes coherent, coordinated care.
  - **Legal responsibilities**: The legal aspect of documentation in medicine.
  - **Communication between healthcare professionals**: Facilitating exchanges and transitions between teams and departments.

2. Key elements of the documentation
- **Identification data**: Basic information about the patient.
- **Initial assessment**: Initial observations, symptoms, vital signs.
- **Care plan**: Planned interventions, objectives, treatments.
- **Progress and follow-up**: Regular updates on the patient's condition and response to treatment.
- **Special notes**: Allergies, advance directives, important decisions.
- **Transfers and discharges**: Information to be shared during a transition of care.

3. Confidentiality principles
- **Respect for patients' rights**: the right to privacy and security of personal information.
- **Regulations and standards**: Local and national legislation, ethical standards.
- **Consequences of a breach**: legal, ethical and professional implications.

4. Information management
- **Secure storage**: Protecting physical files and electronic systems.
- **Limited access**: Ensure that only authorised professionals have access to the data.
- **Information transmission**: Secure data sharing between professionals and establishments.
- **Data destruction**: Procedures for the correct disposal of sensitive information.

5. Specific challenges in acute medicine
- **Emergencies and confidentiality**: Managing privacy in time-critical situations.
- **Large teams**: Co-ordination between multiple stakeholders while respecting confidentiality.
- **Patients unable to consent**: How to protect their information in the absence of explicit consent.

6. Consent and information sharing
- **Obtaining informed consent**: Explaining why and how the information will be used.
- **Exceptional situations**: When and how to disclose information without consent.
- **Families and friends**: Navigating communication while respecting patients' rights.

7. Training and updates
- **Keeping up to date**: legislative developments, technologies, best practice.
- **Ongoing training**: Workshops, seminars, certifications.
- **Feedback**: Learning from past mistakes to improve future practices.

8. Self-evaluation and audits
- **Internal audits**: Ensuring compliance with documentation and confidentiality standards.
- **Constructive feedback**: Using audits to identify areas for improvement.
- **Interdisciplinary collaboration**: Working together to strengthen practices.

Documentation and confidentiality are cornerstones of nursing practice, particularly in acute medicine. Meticulous attention to these aspects not only ensures quality care, but also reinforces mutual trust and respect between the patient and the nursing team.

Chapter 7.
TOOLS AND TECHNOLOGIES IN ACUTE MEDICINE

Monitors and machines vital monitoring

In acute medicine, closely monitoring a patient's vital signs can mean the difference between life and death. Nurses are often on the front line of this monitoring, linking the patient to sophisticated technical devices. These machines, while essential, require a thorough understanding of how they work, how to interpret the data they provide, and appropriate interventions based on this data.

1. Introduction to vital signs monitoring
   * **Why monitor**: The importance of continuous monitoring in acute medicine.
   * **History and development**: From manual palpation to advanced technology.
2. Cardiac monitors
   * **Electrocardiogram (ECG)**: Understanding the waves, intervals, and their meanings.
   * **Recognising arrhythmias**: Identifying and responding to common cardiac arrhythmias.
   * **Temporary pacemakers**: Use, monitoring and potential problems.
3. Blood pressure monitors
   * **Non-invasive measurement (NIM)**: Automatic sphygmomanometers and their applications.
   * **Invasive measurement**: arterial catheters, indications, potential complications.

4. Monitoring oxygenation
- **Pulse oximetry**: Principles, advantages and limitations.
- **Blood gas analysis**: Understanding PaO_2, SaO_2, $PaCO_2$ and their importance.
- **Capnography**: Exhaled CO_2 monitoring, indications and interpretation.

5. Respiratory monitoring
- **Respiratory rate monitors**: Technology, accuracy and common problems.
- **Fans**: Modes, parameters, alarms and common faults.

6. Temperature monitoring
- **Thermistors and thermocouples**: How they work and where they are placed.
- **Hypothermia and hyperthermia**: Recognising, understanding and intervening.

7. Other monitoring systems
- ICP (intracranial pressure) monitors: indications, reading and procedures.
- **Cardiac output:** Measurement methods, interpretation and clinical implications.
- **Monitoring urine flow**: bladder catheters, importance of urine flow in acute medicine.

8. Alarms and alarm management
- **The importance of alarms**: why they exist and when they go off.
- **Alarm-related fatigue**: Phenomenon, consequences and mitigation strategies.
- **Configuration and customisation**: Set the alarm thresholds according to the patient's needs.

9. Maintenance and troubleshooting
- **Daily checks**: Routine checks to ensure that equipment is working properly.
- **Common problems**: Signs of malfunction and basic troubleshooting steps.

- **When to call in a technician**: Recognise the limits of nursing intervention.
10. Ethics and technology
   - **Dependence on technology**: Striking a balance between confidence in the machine and clinical assessment.
   - **Respect for the patient**: Guaranteeing dignity and confidentiality despite constant surveillance.
   - **Ongoing training**: The need to keep abreast of technological developments.

Vital monitoring is an essential component of care in acute medicine. Nurses need to master these tools to provide safe and effective care, while keeping the patient in mind behind every trace, every number and every alarm.

The use of defibrillators and temporary pacemakers

Temporary defibrillators and pacemakers are crucial devices in the management of cardiac emergencies. These devices can restore heart rhythm and save lives in critical situations. Although essential, they require in-depth knowledge on the part of nurses if they are to be used safely and effectively.

1. Introduction to defibrillation and cardiac stimulation
   - **Definition and basic principles**: Understand what defibrillation and cardiac stimulation are.
   - **Indications**: Recognise the situations in which these devices are needed.
2. Defibrillators
   - **How it works**: Understanding the technology behind defibrillation.

- **Types of defibrillator**: Automatic External Defibrillator (AED), semi-automatic and manual.
- **Electrodes and placement**: Importance of location and correct technique.
- **Resuscitation protocols**: Cardiac resuscitation algorithm and the role of defibrillation.
- **Maintenance and inspection**: Ensure that the appliance is in good working order.

3. Temporary pacemakers
- **Why a temporary pacemaker**: Clinical indications and benefits.
- **How it works**: Basic principles of cardiac stimulation.
- **Insertion**: Transcutaneous versus transvenous route.
- **Settings and parameters**: Understanding modes, thresholds and other parameters.
- **Complications and management**: Recognising and dealing with common complications.

4. Interface with other devices
- **Interaction with cardiac monitors**: Interpretation of ECG tracings when using a pacemaker.
- **Simultaneous use with other devices**: Combination with implantable defibrillators, for example.

5. Special situations
- **Defibrillation in special patients**: children, pregnant women, patients with implantable cardiac devices.
- **Post-operative temporary pacemakers**: Indications and management after cardiac surgery.

6. Ethical and legislative aspects
- **Informed consent**: Ensuring that the patient or his or her family understands the procedure.
- **End-of-life decisions and resuscitation**: Respect the patient's wishes regarding resuscitation.
- **Professional responsibilities**: Knowing the legal limits and responsibilities associated with the use of these devices.

7. Training and skills
  - **Importance of ongoing training**: Keeping up to date with technological and clinical developments.
  - **Simulations and workshops**: The importance of regular practice to maintain skills.
  - **Certifications**: Obtaining and renewing the certifications required to use these devices.
8. Conclusion and outlook
  - **Future developments**: Technological advances in defibrillation and cardiac stimulation.
  - **Central role of the nurse**: To emphasise the importance of the nurse in the management of cardiac emergencies and the management of these devices.

The effective use of temporary defibrillators and pacemakers requires both technical expertise and clinical sensitivity. Nurses, as the backbone of acute care, play a vital role in ensuring that these devices are used optimally and safely, while respecting patients' needs and rights.

Technological innovations : telemedicine portable devices

In the digital age, medicine is evolving at breakneck speed, profoundly changing clinical practices and the landscape of care. From virtual consultations to wearable monitoring devices, technological innovations promise more accessible, personalised and efficient medicine. Nurses, key players in the healthcare system, are at the forefront of this revolution.

1. Telemedicine: definition and scope
  - **What is telemedicine**: An introduction to the basic concepts.

- **Advantages and disadvantages**: The weight of technology versus human interaction.
- **The different forms**: From teleconsultation to remote monitoring.

2. Teleconsultation
- **How it works**: How does a remote consultation work?
- **Tools and platforms**: The technologies behind teleconsultation.
- **Limits and challenges**: Situations where physical presence is essential.

3. Wearable devices and healthcare applications
- **Connected watches and bracelets**: Monitoring heart rate, physical activity, sleep...
- **Medical monitoring applications**: diabetes management, blood pressure monitoring, medication reminders, etc.
- **Implications for nurses**: How can these data be integrated into patient monitoring?

4. Remote medical monitoring
- **Home devices**: heart monitors, blood pressure monitors, connected spirometers, etc.
- **Data transmission and analysis**: How are data sent and interpreted by healthcare professionals?
- **Remote intervention**: Actions can be carried out without a physical presence.

5. Virtual and augmented reality in healthcare
- **Therapeutic applications**: Pain treatment, cognitive therapies, rehabilitation, etc.
- **Medical and nursing training**: simulations, emergency scenarios, virtual anatomy...

6. Artificial intelligence (AI) and robotics
- **AI in diagnostics**: diagnostic assistance, interpretation of medical images.
- **Robot assistants**: Helping with care, transporting equipment, interacting with patients.

- **Ethics and AI**: What are the limits for the machine in medicine?
7. The importance of data security
   - **Protection of personal data**: regulations and best practice.
   - **Cybersecurity**: Protecting patient information from external threats.
8. Ethical aspects of health technologies
   - **Equity of access**: Do all patients have access to these technologies?
   - The care-giver-patient relationship in the digital age: preserving the humanity of care.
9. Implications for nursing education
   - Integrating technology into curricula: training future nurses in these tools.
   - **Ongoing training**: Keeping up to date with rapidly evolving technologies.
10. Conclusion and outlook
   - Technology as an ally, not a replacement: Keeping people at the heart of medicine.
   - **Future challenges**: Anticipating future developments and their implications for nursing practice.

While technology is transforming medicine, it is the combination of these innovative tools with the expertise, compassion and humanity of nurses that will make the difference. These innovations promise to deliver more proactive, preventative and personalised care, while emphasising collaboration and communication between carers and patients.

Chapter 8.
COMMON MEDICINES
AND ADMINISTRATION

Essential drug classes in acute medicine

Acute medicine often requires rapid and effective interventions to treat or stabilise patients. Medicines play a crucial role in this. Nurses must have in-depth knowledge of the essential drug classes commonly used in acute medicine to ensure safe and optimal administration.

1. Introduction
   - The importance of pharmacology in acute medicine
   - The nurse's role in administering and monitoring medicines
2. Analgesics
   - **Opiates**: Morphine, Fentanyl, Oxycodone...
   - Non-steroidal anti-inflammatory drugs (NSAIDs): Ibuprofen, Naproxen, etc.
   - Paracetamol (Acetaminophen)
3. Cardiovascular drugs
   - **Anti-arrhythmics**: Amiodarone, Lidocaine...
   - **Antihypertensive agents**: beta-blockers, diuretics, ACE inhibitors, etc.
   - **Vasopressors**: Adrenaline (Epinephrine), Noradrenaline (Norepinephrine)...
4. Respiratory drugs
   - **Bronchodilators**: Salbutamol, Ipratropium...
   - **Inhaled steroids**: Budesonide, Fluticasone...
   - Leukotriene antagonists: Montelukast...
5. Neurological drugs
   - **Anticonvulsants**: Diazepam, Phenytoin...
   - Sedatives and anxiolytics: Midazolam, Lorazepam...

6. Gastrointestinal medicines
   - **Antiemetics**: Metoclopramide, Ondansetron...
   - **Antiulcer drugs**: Omeprazole, Ranitidine...
7. Antibiotics and antivirals
   - Cephalosporins, penicillins, macrolides...
   - Antiretrovirals for severe infections: Oseltamivir...
8. Metabolic and endocrine medicines
   - Insulins and oral antidiabetics: Metformin, Glibenclamide...
   - Thyroid and anti-thyroid hormones: Levothyroxine, Propylthiouracil...
9. Resuscitation agents
   - **Adrenergic agonists**: Adrenalin, Noradrenalin...
   - **Antagonists**: Naloxone for opioid overdoses...
10. Haematological drugs
    - **Anticoagulants**: Heparin, Warfarin...
    - Antiplatelet agents: Aspirin, Clopidogrel, etc.
11. Electrolytes and substitutes
    - Salt solutions, Potassium, Sodium bicarbonate...
12. Conclusion
    - **Secure administration**: double-checking, error prevention.
    - **Monitoring side effects**: Knowledge of drug interactions, signs of overdose or allergic reactions.

Medicines are a vital component of acute medical interventions. Nurses, through their training and experience, are ideally placed to administer these drugs safely, monitor their effects, and educate patients on their use. A thorough knowledge of essential drug classes and their clinical implications is therefore essential to ensure optimal patient care.

Principles of administration and surveillance

Administering medicines in acute medicine is a crucial skill for nurses. With the potential to cause harm or even fatal consequences, accurate administration and careful monitoring are imperative. Understanding the fundamental principles of administration and monitoring ensures that patients receive the safest and most effective care possible.

1. Introduction
   - The importance of secure administration
   - The relationship between administration and supervision
2. The five essentials of drug administration
   - **Good patient**: Check the patient's identity before administration.
   - **Good medicine**: Checking the label, the medicine prescribed and its integrity.
   - **Correct dose**: Check the prescribed and prepared doses.
   - **Correct route**: Ensure the appropriate route of administration (oral, IV, IM, etc.).
   - **Right time**: Respect for the patient's schedule and specific needs.
3. Administration techniques
   - **Oral**: tablets, liquids, capsules...
   - **Injectable**: Intravenous, intramuscular, subcutaneous...
   - **Topical**: creams, gels, patches, etc.
   - **Inhalation**: Aerosols, powder devices, etc.
4. Control and double-checking
   - **High-risk drugs**: Heparin, insulin, anaesthetic drugs, etc.

- Procedures for double checking: When and how to perform.

5. Post-administration monitoring
   - **Expected therapeutic effects**: Recognising when the drug has the desired effect.
   - **Common side effects**: Know what to look for depending on the medicine you are taking.
   - **Signs of overdose**: Specific symptoms to watch for.

6. Drug interactions
   - **Knowledge of common drugs that interact**: for example, anticoagulants with certain antibiotics.
   - **Potential consequences of interactions**: Adverse reactions, reduced efficacy, etc.

7. Patient education
   - **Explain the medicine**: what it does and why it is used.
   - **Possible side effects**: Inform the patient of what to expect.
   - **Adherence to treatment**: Advice to help the patient follow the therapeutic regime.

8. Documentation
   - **The importance of precise documentation**: who, what, when, how and why.
   - **Incident reports**: When and how to report an error or an undesirable event.

9. Other considerations
   - **Cultural considerations**: Respect patients' specific beliefs and needs.
   - **Patients with special needs**: Children, the elderly, the disabled, etc.

10. Conclusion
    - The importance of constantly updating our knowledge: ongoing training, seminars, workshops.

Nurses are often the last link in the chain between the drug prescription and the patient. Appropriate administration and rigorous monitoring are essential to ensure not only the effectiveness of the treatment, but also the safety of the patient. Understanding and mastering these fundamental principles ensures that the care provided is of the highest possible quality.

Managing adverse reactions and drug interactions

Adverse drug reactions and interactions are major concerns for healthcare professionals in acute medicine. These incidents can compromise the effectiveness of treatment, increase morbidity and even, in serious cases, lead to death. Nurses are on the front line in identifying, managing and preventing these events.

1. Introduction
   - Definition of adverse reactions and drug interactions
   - The importance of early detection and treatment
2. Understanding opposing reactions
   - **Types of reaction**: Allergic, toxic, idiosyncratic...
   - **Identifying symptoms**: Skin rashes, breathing difficulties, heart problems...
   - **Rapid intervention**: First aid, antidotes, emergency protocols...
3. Drug interactions: understanding the mechanisms
   - **Pharmacodynamic interactions**: Two drugs with similar or opposite effects.
   - **Pharmacokinetic interactions**: Changes in absorption, metabolism, distribution or excretion.
   - **Food interactions**: Foods that may alter the effect of a medicine.
4. Identify patients at risk
   - **Polymedication**: Increased risk in patients taking several medications.

- **Special populations**: Elderly people, children, pregnant women, etc.
- **Concomitant medical conditions**: Hepatic or renal insufficiency, heart disease...

5. Preventing drug interactions
- **Complete medication review**: On admission, when there are changes in treatment.
- **Use of software and databases**: to help detect and prevent potential interactions.
- **Patient education**: Informing patients about the risks and signs of interactions.

6. Management of identified interactions
- **Adaptation of treatment**: Change of medication, adjustment of dosage.
- **Increased monitoring**: monitoring of vital parameters and blood tests.
- **Documentation and communication**: Informing the medical team, the patient and the family.

7. Continuing education and training for nurses
- **Regular updates**: New drugs, new interactions.
- **Simulation scenarios**: practising responses to different situations.
- **Interprofessional exchange**: learning from the experience and knowledge of colleagues.

8. The importance of the declaration
- **Reporting systems**: Notifying health authorities of adverse reactions and interactions.
- **Learning from mistakes**: Analysing incidents to avoid repeating them.

9. Conclusion
- **The crucial role of the nurse**: detection, intervention, education.
- Importance of close collaboration with the medical team: teamwork for patient safety.

Managing adverse drug reactions and interactions is an essential part of nursing practice in acute medicine. By remaining informed, vigilant and proactive, nurses can make a major contribution to the safety and effectiveness of patient treatment.

Chapter 9.
MANAGEMENT OF INTRAVENOUS ACCESS LINES

Types of catheter and indications

Catheters are medical devices commonly used in medicine for a variety of reasons. Their choice depends on the clinical indication, the desired duration of use and the anatomical access required. Here is an overview of the different types of catheter and their main indications.

1. Introduction
   - Definition of a catheter
   - Importance of choosing the right catheter for the right indication
2. Peripheral venous catheters (PVC)
   - **Description**: Short tubes inserted into a peripheral vein, often on the arm.
   - **Indications**: Short-term administration of drugs, fluids, transfusions, blood sampling.
   - **Limitations**: Risk of venous irritation with certain medicines.
3. Central venous catheters (CVC)
   - **Description**: Longer tubes inserted into a major vein, often the internal jugular, subclavian or femoral vein.
   - **Indications**: Administration of irritant drugs, total parenteral nutrition, long-term access.
     - Special types:
     - Hickman/Broviac catheter: For prolonged use.
     - **Port-a-Cath (PAC)**: Implanted under the skin for long-term use.

- **Swan-Ganz catheter (pulmonary catheter)**: Measurement of cardiac and pulmonary pressures.

4. Arterial catheters
   - **Description**: Inserted into an artery, often the radial or femoral artery.
   - **Indications**: Continuous blood pressure monitoring, arterial blood sampling.

5. Urinary catheters (bladder catheters)
   - **Description**: Tubes inserted into the bladder via the urethra.
   - **Indications**: Urinary retention, urine flow monitoring, surgical procedures.
      - Types:
      - **Indwelling probe**: For long-term use.
      - **Nelaton probe**: For point drainage.
      - **Foley catheter**: Has a balloon to hold the catheter in place.

6. Epidural and spinal catheters
   - **Description**: Inserted into the epidural or intrathecal space of the spinal column.
   - **Indications**: Anaesthesia, administration of analgesic drugs.

7. Haemodialysis catheters
   - **Description**: Large bore tubing for the rapid blood flow required for dialysis.
   - **Indications**: Haemodialysis, haemofiltration.

8. Suction catheters
   - **Description**: Used to aspirate secretions.
   - **Indications**: Bronchial suction, drainage of fluid collections.

9. Feeding catheters
   - **Description**: Inserted into the stomach or intestine.
   - **Indications**: Long-term enteral feeding.
      - Types:
      - **Gastrostomy**: tube inserted directly into the stomach.

- **Jejunostomy**: tube inserted into the jejunum.
10. Conclusion
- **Importance of appropriate choice**: Ensuring safe and effective treatment.
- **Maintenance and care**: Preventing infections and complications.

Understanding the different types of catheter and their indications is essential for healthcare professionals in order to ensure the best possible patient care while minimising the associated risks.

Potential complications and their management

The use of catheters, although common and often vital in medicine, is not without risks. Nurses need to be aware of these potential complications and know how to manage them effectively.

1. Introduction
- Importance of catheter monitoring
- Prevention as the first step
2. Infectious complications
- **Local infections**: Redness, swelling, pus at the insertion site.
- **Management**: catheter removal, microbial cultures, administration of antibiotics.
- **Bacteremia and septicaemia**: Infection that spreads through the bloodstream.
- **Management**: Catheter removal, systemic antibiotics, management of septic shock.
3. Mechanical complications
- **Catheter obstruction**: Decreased flow, inability to withdraw or inject fluids.

- **Management**: Washing with appropriate solutions, sometimes removal and replacement of catheter.
- **Rupture or leakage**: Leakage of fluids outside the catheter.
- **Management**: Discontinue use, secure site, replace catheter.
- **Catheter migration**: Displacement of the catheter from its original position.
- **Management**: Confirmation by imaging, repositioning or removal.

4. Thrombotic complications
- **Venous thrombosis**: blood clot formed around the catheter.
- **Management**: anticoagulants, removal of catheter if necessary, prevention by regular washing.
- **Embolism**: Release of a clot into the bloodstream.
- **Management**: anticoagulants, cardiac and pulmonary monitoring.

5. Air-related complications
- **Gas embolism**: Entry of air into the circulation via the catheter.
- **Management**: Left lateral decubitus position and Trendelenburg, administration of oxygen, sometimes aspiration of air through the catheter.

6. Traumatic complications
- **Perforation**: An organ or vessel is perforated when the catheter is inserted.
- **Management**: Catheter removal, close monitoring, surgery if necessary.
- **Haematomas**: Accumulation of blood at the insertion site.
- **Management**: Compression, monitoring of progress, surgical evacuation if necessary.

7. Chemical complications
- **Chemical phlebitis**: Irritation of the vein caused by a medicine or solution.
- **Management**: Stop administration, apply warm compresses, monitor, possibly remove catheter.

8. Neurological complications
- **Nerve damage**: Especially in the case of epidural or spinal catheters.
- **Management**: Catheter removal, monitoring of symptoms, neurological consultation.

9. Preventing complications
- Sterile insertion techniques
- Regular training for medical staff
- Regular monitoring and appropriate care of the insertion site
- Patient education

The complications associated with catheters are varied and require constant vigilance on the part of healthcare professionals. Appropriate training, rigorous technique and continuous monitoring can minimise these risks and guarantee patient safety.

Administration of medicines intravenously

Intravenous (IV) drug administration is common practice in the medical field, particularly in acute situations. It allows the drug to act quickly, but requires in-depth knowledge and special care to avoid complications.

1. Introduction
- **Advantages of the intravenous route**: rapid absorption, precise doses, use of large-volume solutions or irritant drugs.

- **The nurse's responsibilities**: Appropriate selection of the injection site, proper preparation of the medication, monitoring the patient.

2. Types of IV administration
   - **Bolus or direct injection**: rapid administration of a small quantity of medication.
   - **Continuous infusion**: constant and regular administration of medicines or solutions.
   - **Intermittent infusion**: Administration of doses of medication at regular intervals.

3. Preparing the medicine
   - **Checking the prescription**: confirming the dose, drug and route of administration.
   - **Hand hygiene**: Wash hands before handling.
   - **Preparation in a sterile environment**: Use of aseptic techniques to avoid contamination.
   - **Checking the drug**: Expiry, integrity, precipitation or discolouration of the product.

4. Selecting and preparing the injection site
   - **Choice of vein**: Preference for veins on the back of the hand, forearm or elbow.
   - **Site assessment**: Avoid damaged, swollen or painful areas.
   - **Disinfection of the site**: Use an antiseptic in a circular motion from the centre outwards.

5. Inserting the IV line
   - **Aseptic technique**: Wear sterile gloves.
   - **Insertion of the catheter**: At an angle of 15-30 degrees to the skin, adjusting to a less acute angle once in the vein.
   - **Confirmation of position**: Return of blood to the catheter tubing.
   - **Fixing the catheter**: Use sterile, transparent dressings.

6. Drug administration
   - **Checking the infusion rate**: Adjustment according to medical prescription.

- **Monitoring during administration**: Observation for signs of complications, such as infiltration or phlebitis.
- **Rinsing**: After administration, use a saline solution to ensure complete drug delivery and maintain catheter patency.

7. Post-administration monitoring
   - **Observing the effects of the drug**: Signs of efficacy or side effects.
   - **Monitoring the insertion site**: looking for signs of infection, infiltration or irritation.

8. Withdrawal of the IV route
   - Hand hygiene: Before removal.
   - **Gentle removal**: With a continuous movement while applying pressure with a sterile compress.
   - **Dressing**: Apply to the site to prevent bleeding.

9. Complications and their management
   - Phlebitis, infiltration, extravasation, gas embolism, infection.
   - Prevention and intervention.

Intravenous drug administration is an essential skill for nurses working in acute medicine. A thorough understanding of techniques, meticulous preparation and careful monitoring are essential to ensure the safety and efficacy of this form of administration.

Chapter 10.
SUPPORT FOR SPECIFIC PATIENTS

Paediatrics :
the child in an acute situation

Paediatrics is a world of its own in the medical world, marked by its own dynamics, challenges and touching moments. When it comes to caring for a child in an acute situation, every second counts, every decision is crucial, but everything must be done with a gentleness adapted to these particularly vulnerable patients.

It is essential to understand that children are not simply "little adults". Their physiology, anatomy and psychology have specific characteristics that require a tailored approach. For example, their narrower airways can become blocked more easily, and their hearts often beat faster at rest than those of adults. These differences, although subtle, can influence the course of an illness or the response to a treatment.

The first interaction with a child in distress requires a careful assessment, often guided by the ABCDE approach, adapted for paediatrics. While assessing the child's condition, the nurse must be aware of normal paediatric vital signs, which vary considerably according to age. A heart rate that would be considered high for an adult may be completely normal for a child.
One of the most valuable skills in paediatrics is the ability to communicate effectively with children and their families. An infant cannot express pain or discomfort in the same way as a teenager. Similarly, a pre-schooler may be terrified of medical equipment, while an older child may be curious. In every situation, it is essential to reassure, inform

and involve parents, who are often the key to understanding their child's needs and feelings.

Pain, which is omnipresent in the medical environment, takes on a new dimension when it comes to children. It must be assessed with tools adapted to the child's age and treated with a combination of medication and non-medicinal techniques. It is a painful experience for a parent to see their child suffer, and the medical team must work hand in hand with the family to alleviate this pain.

The range of acute paediatric conditions is vast, from common infections such as gastroenteritis or otitis to more serious situations such as trauma or poisoning. Each scenario requires specific knowledge and rapid action.
Administering medication to a child is a delicate exercise. Mistakes can be fatal. The dosage, generally based on the child's weight, must be checked carefully, and each drug administered with caution.

Caring for children in acute situations is a challenge that requires expertise, gentleness and effective communication. In this world where fragility and hope go hand in hand, every healthcare professional plays a crucial role in offering the best to these little patients.

Gerontology :
the elderly patient in acute medicine

In the vast world of medicine, the management of the elderly patient in an acute situation presents its own challenges, nuances and particularities. As the world's population ages, healthcare professionals are increasingly faced with complex situations where the effects of ageing interact with acute conditions, creating a mosaic of symptoms and needs that require a holistic approach.

It is often said that older people are not simply "older adults". Indeed, ageing is accompanied by physiological, anatomical and psychosocial changes that can affect the way a disease manifests itself and progresses. For example, declining kidney function can alter the way a drug is metabolised, while loss of muscle mass can influence an individual's mobility and strength.

One of the major challenges in gerontology is polyspathology. Elderly people often suffer from several chronic illnesses, which may interact with each other or with a new acute condition. A patient may be admitted with pneumonia, but it may be their diabetes or heart disease that complicates the clinical picture. The nurse must then carefully navigate this complex sea of symptoms and medications, seeking to provide optimal care while avoiding complications.

Communication with the elderly patient in an acute situation is also essential. With age, cognitive deficits can appear, making it more difficult to understand or express oneself. It is crucial to approach patients with patience and empathy, and to ensure that they fully understand their situation and the care proposed. Whenever possible, including family members can provide valuable insight into the patient's history, medication and preferences.

One of the most poignant aspects of caring for the elderly patient is the confrontation with finitude. Palliative and end-of-life care must often be considered, seeking to offer maximum quality of life at times when recovery is no longer possible. At these delicate moments, the nurse becomes a pillar, supporting both patient and family, guiding with compassion and professionalism.

Gerontology in acute medicine is above all a matter of the heart and mind. Every patient is a book of stories, memories and lessons. Through the medical and ethical challenges, nurses have the priceless opportunity to offer, even in the darkest moments, a beacon of hope, dignity and respect.

Patients with special needs: disability, mental health, etc.

Navigating the intricacies of acute medicine is a complex task for any healthcare professional. However, when it comes to patients with special needs, this complexity reaches a new level. These individuals, whether affected by a physical, cognitive, sensory or mental health disability, bring with them a unique set of needs and dynamics.

First of all, let's look at the spectrum of disability. A patient with paraplegia, for example, will have different needs to a patient with deafness. The first thing every nurse needs to recognise is the individual behind the disability. Knowledge and familiarity with disability are important, but they must be combined with a patient-centred approach, seeking to understand the patient's needs, wishes and personal experiences.

Patients with mental health problems bring another set of challenges. Conditions such as schizophrenia, bipolar disorder or major depression can influence how patients perceive their acute illness, how they interact with care staff and how they adhere to treatment plans. The nurse must be both vigilant and empathetic, seeking to establish a relationship of trust while ensuring the safety of the patient and the team.

Then there are patients with cognitive impairments, whether dementia, developmental delay or other conditions. These individuals may have difficulty

86

understanding or communicating their symptoms, pain or needs. A patient and individualised approach is crucial, with appropriate communication tools, whether images, gestures or assistive technologies.

Communication is the common thread linking all these special needs. Whether it's an interpreter for a deaf patient, a de-escalation approach for a patient in psychotic crisis, or simply listening attentively to an anxious patient, the nurse's ability to communicate effectively is essential.

Finally, training and education continue to play a crucial role. The world of special needs is vast and constantly changing. Nurses need to stay up to date, seek out specialist training and, above all, learn from every interaction with these patients.

When caring for patients with special needs in acute medicine, the task can seem daunting. However, through the complexity and challenges, there are incredible opportunities for learning, growth and deeply human moments. It is in these interactions that the essence of nursing - compassion, understanding and selflessness - shines brightest.

Chapter 11.
HYGIENE AND PREVENTION INFECTIONS

Principles of hygiene in acute medicine

Hygiene in acute medicine is an absolute priority. In an environment where patients are often vulnerable, with weakened immune systems or suffering from infections, strict hygiene protocols are not only desirable, they are vital. The speed of treatment and the acuity of medical situations amplify the need for impeccable hygiene practices.

One of the first things nurses are taught is the importance of hand washing. Simple on the face of it, this gesture is in fact an essential first line of defence against the spread of infections. Hands, which are in constant contact with patients, medical devices and the environment, are the main vector for the transmission of pathogens. Meticulous hand washing, using appropriate techniques and at key moments (before and after each contact with a patient, after touching potentially contaminated surfaces, etc.), can make all the difference.

Next comes the judicious use of personal protective equipment (PPE). Whether it's gloves, masks, gowns or protective glasses, each item has its place and its time. It's not just to protect the nurse, but also to prevent cross-transmission between patients. Knowing when and how to use them, and above all how to remove them correctly, is essential to guarantee their effectiveness.
Disinfection and sterilisation of equipment are also central to the principles of hygiene. In an acute setting, medical devices such as stethoscopes, monitors and surgical

instruments must be rigorously cleaned and sterilised. Each tool has its own recommendations for disinfection, and it's crucial to follow them to the letter.

The cleanliness of the environment is just as crucial. Floors, surfaces and bedding all need to be regularly cleaned with appropriate disinfectants. Cleaning protocols must be rigorously followed, particularly in high-risk areas such as isolation wards or intensive care units.

Finally, ongoing education and training are essential. Pathogens evolve, as do our knowledge and technologies. Nurses need to be informed about the latest advances, new bacterial or viral strains and the best practices for combating them.

In acute medicine, the urgency and complexity of situations can sometimes give the impression that hygiene is secondary. Yet it is at the heart of the practice. Good hygiene is not just a question of cleanliness; it's a question of safety, quality of care and, ultimately, respect for the patient. In the ceaseless ballet that is acute medicine, hygiene is the silent but essential choreography that ensures the grace and efficiency of every movement.

Prevention of nosocomial infections

Hospital-acquired infections, also known as healthcare-associated infections, represent a major challenge for the medical world. Contracted during a stay in a healthcare facility, they can have serious consequences for patients, ranging from delayed recovery to severe and even fatal complications. In the fast-paced environment of acute medicine, where patients are particularly vulnerable and interactions are frequent, preventing these infections is vital.

Active surveillance is the first step. Setting up an infection surveillance system in each establishment means that any unusual increase in infections can be detected quickly, the sources identified and corrective measures put in place.

Hand washing is, once again, the first line of defence. Using soap and water or a hydro-alcoholic solution at key moments, such as before and after any contact with a patient, is a simple but powerful way of reducing the risk.

The **management of catheters and other invasive devices** is essential. The insertion, maintenance and removal of these devices must follow strict protocols to minimise the risk of infection. Every day, an assessment must be made to determine whether these devices are still needed, as their prolonged presence increases the risk of infection.

Isolators and isolation precautions are also crucial. When a patient is known or suspected to be a carrier of a transmissible infectious agent, isolation measures must be put in place to prevent the spread of infection to other patients, visitors or healthcare staff.

Antimicrobial prophylaxis, when used judiciously, can effectively prevent certain infections. However, its use must be based on sound scientific evidence to avoid overuse and antibiotic resistance.

The **upkeep of the premises** is also fundamental. Cleaning services must follow strict protocols to ensure that rooms are disinfected, especially after a patient has left and before a new one arrives.

Staff **training** is an essential component. All healthcare professionals, whether nurses, doctors or cleaners, must be regularly trained and informed about best practice in infection prevention.

The **involvement of patients and their families** can also play a role. Informing them about basic hygiene measures, such as hand washing, and encouraging them to remind staff to do so, reinforces the culture of prevention.

Finally, an **organisational culture** focused on patient safety is essential. Encouraging the reporting of incidents, without fear of reprimand, and adopting a continuous improvement approach are essential to reducing hospital-acquired infections.

Preventing nosocomial infections is a responsibility shared by all those involved in the healthcare chain. It's a daily commitment, where every gesture counts, and requires constant vigilance. In this battle, anticipation, training and rigour are our best allies.

Importance of vaccination for staff

Vaccinating healthcare staff is a major public health and patient safety issue. Healthcare professionals are on the front line when it comes to infectious diseases, and are therefore more exposed to the risk of contamination. What's more, they are in constant contact with patients who are often vulnerable, which puts them at the heart of a potential transmission dynamic. Vaccinating staff is not just about individual protection; it is part of a collective strategy to defend against epidemics.

- **Personal protection:** Healthcare professionals are exposed to a variety of pathogens. Getting vaccinated reduces their risk of contracting vaccine-preventable diseases, thereby ensuring their own health and their ability to continue working effectively.
- **Reduced transmission:** A vaccinated healthcare professional is less likely to transmit a disease to his or her patients, colleagues or own family. This is particularly crucial for at-risk patients, such as neonates, the elderly or immunocompromised people, who may develop serious forms of certain diseases.

- **Preventing epidemics:** In a hospital environment, population density and proximity to patients encourage the rapid spread of infections. Ensuring high vaccination coverage among staff reduces the risk of epidemics within the establishment.
- **Role model:** Healthcare professionals play an exemplary role in society. When they are vaccinated, they send a strong message to the public about the importance and safety of vaccination. Their support for vaccination programmes strengthens public confidence.
- **Savings for the healthcare system:** Vaccine-preventable diseases can lead to absence from work, prolonged hospitalisation and complications, all of which generate additional costs for the healthcare system. By vaccinating healthcare workers, these costs can be avoided.
- **Ethical obligation:** Beyond the pragmatic arguments, there is an ethical dimension to the vaccination of healthcare staff. The Hippocratic oath states "First, do no harm". By being vaccinated, healthcare professionals are putting this principle into action, by ensuring that they are not a vector of disease for their patients.
- **Protection against new risks:** Medicine and pathogens are constantly evolving. With the emergence of new diseases and the resurgence of old ones, it is crucial that healthcare staff are protected and up to date with vaccination recommendations.

Vaccinating healthcare staff is both an individual and collective initiative, essential to ensuring patient safety, the peace of mind of professionals and the robustness of the healthcare system. In a world where infectious threats are constantly evolving, vaccination remains one of our most effective and reliable tools.

Chapter 12.
THE ROLE OF THE NURSE
PRACTITIONER IN ACUTE MEDICINE

Training and qualifications
the nurse practitioner

Nurse practitioners, sometimes called "specialised clinical nurses" or "specialised nurse practitioners" depending on the country, are healthcare professionals with advanced training and broad clinical expertise. They are capable of making diagnoses, prescribing treatments, initiating additional examinations and playing an active part in the overall management of patients, often in close collaboration with doctors and other healthcare professionals. The nurse practitioner's training and qualification pathway is demanding and adapted to these extensive responsibilities.

- **Initial nursing training:** The first step in becoming a nurse practitioner is to obtain a degree in nursing. This is usually done as part of a three- to four-year university programme, leading to a bachelor's or bachelor's degree in nursing.
- **Clinical experience:** Before you can enrol in a nurse practitioner programme, you are often required to have several years of clinical experience as a nurse. This experience provides practical skills and a thorough understanding of patient care.
- **Advanced   training:** Nurse practitioner training is generally at Master's level or equivalent. It generally lasts two years, although the duration may vary depending on the country and speciality. This training

includes advanced theoretical courses, research work and intensive clinical training under supervision.

- **Specialisation:** Depending on the country and the institution, it is possible to specialise in areas such as paediatrics, geriatrics, psychiatry, acute care, women's health, etc. These specialities often require additional training and specific clinical placements. These specialities often require additional training and specific clinical placements.
- **Certification:** After completing their training, nurse practitioners are often required to pass a certification examination to prove their skills. Certification is often recognised by national or regional bodies and may require periodic renewal, often combined with continuing education.
- **Maintaining skills:** Medicine is constantly evolving. Nurse practitioners are therefore required to take regular continuing education courses to keep their skills up to date and meet re-certification requirements.
- **Legislation and regulatory framework:** The roles and responsibilities of nurse practitioners can vary considerably between countries and regions. It is essential to be informed and to respect the regulatory framework in force.

The training and qualifications of nurse practitioners are designed to guarantee optimal patient care. These professionals bring added value to the medical team, particularly in contexts where access to doctors is limited or in specific specialties. They represent an essential link in the healthcare system, combining clinical competence, decision-making capacity and proximity to patients.

Scope of skills and practice

The nurse practitioner (NP) is a key professional in medical care, acting as a bridge between traditional nurses and doctors. Their scope of skills and practice is vast, adapted to the complex needs of modern healthcare systems. As highly qualified clinicians, NPs have the expertise to act both independently and in collaboration with other specialists.

- **Advanced clinical assessment:** IPs are trained to carry out comprehensive clinical assessments, including medical history-taking, physical examination, symptom interpretation and assessment of the patient's psychosocial needs.
- **Diagnosis:** In many countries, IPs have the right to make diagnoses, to identify illnesses, disorders or diseases on the basis of the symptoms presented by the patient.
- **Prescription: Depending on** local regulations, the PI may have the right to prescribe medicines, treatments or therapies, as well as order diagnostic tests such as blood tests, X-rays or ultrasounds.
- **Medical procedures:** Some IPs are trained to carry out specific medical procedures, such as sutures, biopsies, intubations or catheter insertion.
- **Referral and collaboration:** The IP is often a central point of liaison between the patient and other specialists. They can refer the patient to other professionals for specialist care, while ensuring consistent follow-up care.
- **Education and health promotion:** As well as providing direct care, IPs play a crucial role in educating patients, helping them to understand their condition and the treatments on offer, and encouraging them to adopt healthy behaviours.

- **Research and evaluation:** Many PIs are involved in clinical research, helping to improve medical practice and evaluate new interventions.
- **Management and leadership:** within healthcare establishments, PIs may occupy management positions, supervising teams, participating in strategic planning or implementing healthcare policies.
- **Specialisations:** Like doctors, IPs can specialise in specific fields, such as cardiology, paediatrics, psychiatry or geriatrics, to name but a few.
- **Consultation and mentoring:** With their experience and expertise, NPs often act as mentors for younger nurses or other healthcare professionals, guiding their professional development.

Nurse practitioners occupy a prominent place in the spectrum of medical care, providing advanced expertise while maintaining a patient-centred approach. The constant evolution of the medical field makes their role even more crucial, as they can quickly adapt to the changing needs of patients and healthcare systems.

Working with doctors and other specialists

At the heart of multidisciplinary medical teams, the nurse practitioner (NP) works closely with doctors, surgeons, pharmacists, therapists, social workers and other specialists. The aim of this collaboration is to ensure that patients receive optimum, holistic care, drawing on the complementary skills of each professional.

- **Effective communication:** One of the keys to successful collaboration is the ability to communicate clearly and effectively. This involves sharing relevant information about the patient's condition, discussing

96

possible diagnoses and treatment options, and ensuring that the patient is at the centre of all decisions.

- **Understanding roles:** Each member of the team has a unique set of skills and responsibilities. Understanding each person's limitations and areas of expertise means that patients can be directed to the right specialist at the right time.
- **Regular consultation:** Team meetings, clinical rounds and case conferences are ideal opportunities to discuss complex cases, exchange views and draw up coordinated care plans.
- **Mutual respect:** Recognition of the value of each professional fosters an atmosphere of mutual respect, which is essential for harmonious collaboration. Everyone must feel valued and listened to.
- **Interprofessional training:** More and more healthcare institutions are promoting interprofessional training, where different specialists learn side by side, reinforcing collaboration right from the start of their careers.
- **Technology and shared medical records:** The use of shared electronic medical records facilitates collaboration by enabling all the professionals involved to access the necessary information in real time.
- **Coordination of care:** With its global approach, the nurse practitioner can play a coordinating role, ensuring continuity of care and making sure that the patient receives the necessary interventions from all specialists.
- **Ethical reflection:** Collaboration can also involve ethical discussions, particularly when it comes to making difficult decisions about treatment or end-of-life care.
- **Continuing professional development:** IPs, like other healthcare professionals, need to keep abreast

of medical advances. Taking part in joint training courses or conferences with other specialists enriches everyone's perspective.

• **Mutual support:** The medical field can be stressful. Having a close-knit team, where each member supports the others, is essential for the well-being of the professionals and the quality of the care offered.

Collaboration between the nurse practitioner and other specialists is a cornerstone of modern healthcare. It ensures that patients benefit from a collective expertise, providing comprehensive care tailored to their needs. In this collaborative environment, each professional makes his or her own contribution, and together they work towards the optimum well-being of the patient.

Chapter 13.
PREVENTION AND EDUCATION OF PATIENTS

Educating people about risk factors

One of the fundamental missions of healthcare professionals, particularly nurse practitioners, is to educate patients, their families and the community about the risk factors associated with various medical conditions. This proactive education can prevent many complications and promote a healthy lifestyle.

- **Definition and importance:** A risk factor is any characteristic or exposure of an individual that increases the likelihood of developing an illness or injury. Understanding these factors enables preventive strategies to be put in place.
- **Modifiable and non-modifiable risk factors:** While some factors, such as age or genetics, cannot be modified, others, such as lifestyle or environment, can be adjusted to reduce risk.
- **Risk assessment:** Nurses need to know how to assess the specific risks for each patient, based on their history, lifestyle and genetics.
- Education strategies:
    - **Open dialogue:** Engaging in honest conversations with patients, listening to their concerns and providing factual information.
    - **Teaching materials:** Provide brochures, videos or other resources to help patients understand their risks.

- **Workshops and seminars:** Organise educational sessions on specific themes, such as diet, exercise or stress management.
- Common risk factors and their management:
    - **Smoking:** Informing people about the dangers of smoking and providing resources for quitting.
    - **Unbalanced diet:** Promote a balanced diet rich in fruit, vegetables, whole grains and lean proteins.
    - **Sedentary lifestyle:** Encourage regular physical activity suited to the patient's age and physical condition.
    - **Excessive alcohol consumption:** Discuss the recommended limits and dangers of excessive alcohol consumption.
    - **Stress:** Offer stress management techniques such as meditation or relaxation.
- **Raising awareness of prevention:** A reminder of the importance of regular medical check-ups, screening and vaccinations to prevent disease.
- **Collaboration with other professionals:** Working with dieticians, physiotherapists, psychologists or other specialists to provide comprehensive care.
- **Follow-up and reassessment:** Since risk factors and lifestyles can change over time, it is essential to review these factors with the patient on a regular basis.
- **Community involvement:** Participating in public health events or initiatives to raise community awareness of common risk factors and their management.

Educating people about risk factors is an investment in their future well-being. By providing accurate information and offering resources and support, nurses can make a significant contribution to disease prevention and the promotion of a healthy lifestyle.

Encouraging healthy behaviour

Promoting healthy behaviour is a cornerstone of prevention in medicine. While acute medicine often focuses on treating urgent conditions, encouraging healthy behaviours can prevent these emergencies from occurring in the first place. Nurses, as trusted intermediaries between the healthcare system and patients, play an essential role in this respect.

- Understanding the patient:
  - **Active listening:** Taking the time to listen to the patient's concerns, needs and obstacles.
  - **Assessment of current habits:** Identify where the patient is in their health pathway, including eating habits, physical activity levels, substance use behaviours, etc.
- Education and awareness-raising:
  - **Information:** Provide factual, up-to-date information on the benefits of healthy behaviours.
  - **Myths and misinformation:** Demystifying common misconceptions and providing evidence-based information.
- Motivational strategies:
  - **Motivational interviewing:** Using this technique to help patients recognise and overcome their resistance to change.
  - **Setting goals:** Helping patients to define realistic and measurable goals for their healthy behaviours.

- Promoting a balanced diet:
    - **Knowledge of food groups:** Encouraging a varied diet.
    - **Reading labels:** educating people about the importance of understanding nutritional information.
    - **Cooking at home:** Promote the benefits of preparing meals at home, and provide healthy recipes where possible.
- Encouraging physical exercise:
    - **Benefits of physical activity:** Remind people of the benefits to the body and mind.
    - **Finding a suitable activity:** Helping patients to find an activity that suits them, whether it's walking, dancing, yoga, etc.
- Stress management:
    - **Recognising triggers:** Helping patients to identify what is causing stress in their lives.
    - **Relaxation techniques:** Introduce methods such as meditation, deep breathing and visualisation.
- Avoidance of harmful substances:
    - **Smoking:** providing resources to help people stop smoking.
    - **Alcohol consumption:** Discuss safe limits and the risks associated with excessive consumption.
- Promoting restful sleep:
    - **Sleep hygiene:** advice on the importance of a regular sleep routine and an environment conducive to rest.
- Support networks:
    - **Support groups:** Refer patients to local or online support groups.
    - **Family and friends:** Encourage patients to share their goals with family and friends for support.

- Follow-up:
    - Plan follow-up meetings to discuss progress, overcome obstacles and readjust objectives if necessary.

Encouraging healthy behaviours is not just about imparting information, but about building a relationship of trust with the patient, understanding their specific needs and providing them with the tools and support they need to succeed. By adopting this holistic approach, nurses can make a real difference to their patients' lives.

Transition support towards home care

The transition from hospital to home care is a crucial time for patients and their families. It can be a stressful time, full of uncertainty, but also full of hope at the prospect of a return to normality. Nurses play a central role in ensuring that this transition takes place as smoothly and safely as possible.

- Assessment of the situation at home:
    - **Preliminary visit:** A nurse or other healthcare professional can make a home visit to assess the environment and determine any necessary modifications.
    - **Identification of needs:** Recognition of specific medical needs, such as the need for adapted equipment or medication.
- Training for patients and their carers:
    - **Basic skills:** Training patients and carers in essential skills such as administering medication, monitoring vital signs and carrying out basic care.

- **Responding to emergencies:** Providing clear guidelines on what to do in the event of an emergency.
- Coordination with homecare providers:
    - **Establishing contacts:** Putting patients in touch with home nurses, physiotherapists or other specialists as required.
    - **Fluid communication:** Ensuring a smooth transition by communicating clearly with homecare providers about the patient's condition and needs.
- Planning your outing:
    - **Checklist:** Provide a detailed list of the steps to be taken on discharge from hospital.
    - **Follow-up appointments:** Schedule the appointments required for medical follow-up.
- Emotional support:
    - **Support:** Recognising the feelings of fear, anxiety and uncertainty that patients may experience during the transition.
    - **Guidance:** Offer resources such as support groups or therapy to help manage these emotions.
- Post-transition monitoring:
    - **Follow-up calls:** Organise regular telephone calls to make sure that everything is going well at home.
    - **Regular visits:** Plan home visits to assess the situation and adjust the care plan if necessary.
- Medication management:
    - **Up-to-date list:** Ensure that the patient has an up-to-date list of all their medicines, with the appropriate dosages and times.
    - **Organisation:** Advising on the use of pillboxes or applications to monitor medication intake.

- Progress assessment:
    - **Health diary:** Encourage patients to keep a daily health diary to monitor progress and identify any problems.
    - **Rehabilitation:** If necessary, organise rehabilitation sessions to help with physical and mental recovery.
- Resources and community support:
    - **Local services:** Inform patients about the resources available in their community, such as drug delivery services or patient support programmes.
- Preventing readmissions:
    - **Education:** Providing information on the prevention of common complications associated with their condition.
    - **Warning signs:** Educate them about the signs to look out for that could indicate a deterioration in their condition.

The transition to home care is a journey that requires attentive and caring support. Through meticulous planning, appropriate training and ongoing support, nurses can ensure that their patients continue to receive quality care, even outside the hospital environment.

Chapter 14.
REHABILITATION AND FOLLOW-UP CARE

Planning your outing and care coordination

Discharge from hospital is often a moment of relief mixed with anxiety for patients. The prospect of returning to the comfort of their own homes is alluring, but it is also accompanied by uncertainty about the continuity of care. Nurses, with their central role, are ideally placed to ensure a smooth, safe and reassuring transition for patients.

- Preliminary assessment for discharge :
    - **Patient's state of health:** Is the patient stable and fit to leave hospital?
    - **Self-care skills:** Is the patient capable of looking after themselves or will they need assistance?
- Coordination with the medical team :
    - **Multidisciplinary meeting:** Bringing together doctors, nurses, social workers and physiotherapists to draw up an appropriate discharge plan.
    - **Medicines and prescriptions:** Ensure that the patient has all the necessary prescriptions and understands how to use them.
- Patient and family education :
    - **Post-hospitalisation instructions:** Clearly explain the care to be followed, the warning signs and the frequency of medical appointments.

- **Techniques and skills:** Teaching patients and their relatives the necessary skills, such as changing dressings or administering medication.
- Organisation of home   care :
  - **Home services:** If necessary, organise home nursing, physiotherapy or care assistant services.
  - **Medical equipment:** Arrange for the delivery of any necessary equipment, such as medical beds, wheelchairs or oxygen therapy devices.
- Follow-up appointment :
  - **Medical consultations:** Schedule appointments with specialists, GPs or other healthcare professionals.
  - **Tests and examinations :** Organise any additional tests or follow-up required.
- Coordination with social services :
  - **Home support:** If required, provide help with housework, shopping or cooking.
  - **Rehabilitation programmes:** guiding patients towards programmes adapted to their situation, whether physical, psychological or social.
- Exit documents :
  - **Medical summary:** Provide a detailed account of the hospitalisation, the treatment received and recommendations for the future.
  - **Contact details:** Provide a list of useful numbers in case of questions or emergencies.
- Post-hospital follow-up :
  - **Phone calls:** Check in regularly to make sure everything is going well.
  - **Reassessment:** If necessary, review and adjust the initial care plan according to the patient's progress.

Discharge planning and care coordination are essential to ensure patient safety and promote recovery. Using a holistic, patient-centred approach, nurses can ensure that patients receive appropriate care and continue their recovery in the best possible conditions.

Teamwork with therapists and social workers

In the dynamic and often unpredictable world of acute medicine, nurses do not work alone. They work at the heart of a multidisciplinary team made up of doctors, therapists and social workers, each of whom contributes his or her part to ensuring that patients receive comprehensive, individualised care. This inter-professional collaboration is not only essential to meeting the complex needs of patients, but also enriches the practices and vision of each professional.

- Recognising roles and skills :
  - **Therapists:** They may specialise in various fields such as physiotherapy, occupational therapy or respiratory therapy. Their expertise is crucial in helping patients to regain their mobility and independence or to manage respiratory problems.
  - **Social workers:** Their job is to support patients and their families in dealing with the social, emotional and economic challenges associated with illness or hospitalisation.
- Communication and team meetings :
  - **Regular exchanges:** These are opportunities to share observations, concerns and therapeutic objectives for each patient.
  - **Care planning:** Close collaboration ensures that all aspects of the patient's well-being are

taken into account, whether in terms of physical, mental or social health.

- Coordination of operations :
  - **Organising therapies:** Nurses often need to plan their care around therapy sessions to avoid interference and maximise the effectiveness of interventions.
  - **Emotional and social support:** By working closely with social workers, the nurse can ensure that the patient's emotional and social needs are addressed, whether this involves psychological support, home help or administrative procedures.
- Training and continuing education :
  - **Cross-disciplinary workshops:** These are opportunities to share ideas and deepen mutual understanding of each other's roles and responsibilities, while encouraging the exchange of skills.
  - **Clinical cases:** Discussing complex cases together provides an opportunity to learn from each other and refine management strategies.
- Benefits for the patient:
  - **Holistic care:** Thanks to this collaboration, patients benefit from care that encompasses all their needs.
  - **Smooth transition:** Coordination between the various professionals facilitates the transition between hospital and home, ensuring continuity of care.
- Challenges and solutions :
  - **Professional cultural differences:** Each profession has its own culture, jargon and perspectives. It is therefore crucial to promote mutual understanding and respect.
  - **Interprofessional training:** Encouraging training from higher education onwards

familiarises each professional with other disciplines and strengthens collaboration from the start of their career.

Teamwork between nurses, therapists and social workers is a valuable synergy. Together, they can provide patients with comprehensive care that addresses their medical, physical, emotional and social needs.

Home monitoring and prevention rehospitalisation

The transition from hospital to home care is a delicate and crucial moment in a patient's care pathway. Nurses play a pivotal role in ensuring that this transition is smooth and that the patient's needs continue to be met. What's more, a successful transition can prevent re-hospitalisations, which are often distressing for the patient and costly for the healthcare system.

- Pre-discharge assessment :
    - **Patient's state of health:** Before the patient is discharged home, he or she must be thoroughly assessed to ensure that his or her state of health is stable and that he or she will be able to receive the necessary care at home.
    - **Home environment:** An assessment of the patient's environment, including potential risks and available resources, is essential. The occupational therapist, for example, can contribute to this assessment.
- Planning the outing :
    - **Patient and family education:** Nurses ensure that patients and their families are aware of the signs to watch out for, the medicines to take and upcoming appointments.

- **Coordination with healthcare professionals at home:** Before discharge, the nurse contacts home nurses, GPs or any other professional who will be working in the patient's home.
- Follow-up at home :
    - **Regular visits:** Home nursing visits are used to monitor the patient's state of health, administer treatments and assess the need for adjustments.
    - **Telemedicine: Increasingly** used, telemedicine enables patients to be monitored remotely, treatments to be adjusted and a rapid response to any problems.
- Prevention of complications :
    - **Self-management training:** The nurse trains the patient to recognise the signs of a worsening condition and to take appropriate action.
    - **Medication management :** Ensuring proper compliance with treatment is essential to avoid complications.
- Social reintegration :
    - **Return to daily life:** The nurse encourages and supports the patient in resuming their daily activities, whether leisure, professional or social.
    - **Psychological support:** Hospitalisation can be traumatic, and psychological support at home is often beneficial.
- Communication with the hospital team :
    - **Sharing information:** The home care nurse and the hospital nurse regularly exchange information about the patient's progress, treatment adjustments or potential complications.

111

- **Return to hospital: In the** event of a major complication, the home care nurse coordinates with the hospital to organise a rapid and effective return to hospital.

Follow-up at home is an essential stage in the overall care of the patient. A well-prepared transition, effective coordination with healthcare professionals at home and ongoing support can prevent complications and ensure the best possible quality of life for the patient.

Chapter 15.
CRISIS MANAGEMENT SKILLS

Basic principles of crisis management

Crisis management is an essential part of the nursing role, especially in acute medicine, where situations can evolve rapidly and unpredictably. Approaching a crisis with skill, confidence and empathy can make the difference between a positive outcome and tragic consequences. The fundamental principles of crisis management can help to navigate these situations with discernment.

- Anticipation and preparation :
    - **Ongoing training:** Regular education and updating of knowledge of emergency protocols and best practice are crucial.
    - **Crisis planning:** Having clear protocols in place for various crisis situations, from cardiac decompensation to managing behavioural problems.
- Fast, accurate assessment:
    - **Recognising the signs:** Quickly detecting the warning signs or symptoms of a crisis situation.
    - **Assessing needs:** quickly identifying what the patient needs and what resources are required to meet those needs.
- Effective communication :
    - **Clear and concise:** In a crisis situation, every second counts. Information must be relayed clearly and quickly.
    - **Active listening:** Listening carefully to the patient, their family and the medical team to understand the situation as a whole.

- Adapted intervention :
  - **Act quickly:** Make informed decisions and act quickly to stabilise the patient or the situation.
  - **Remain calm: The** nurse's calm can reassure the patient and the team, even at the most tense moments.
- Emotional support :
  - **Empathy:** Recognising and validating the feelings of patients and their families.
  - **Reassurance:** Reassure the patient about the measures taken and clearly explain the interventions.
- Post-crisis evaluation :
  - **Debrief:** Bring the team together to discuss what went well and areas for improvement.
  - **Emotional support:** Recognising potential post-traumatic stress in patients, families and the medical team and providing appropriate support.
- Continuous improvement:
  - **Feedback:** Using crisis experience to improve protocols and training.
  - **Ongoing training: Keeping abreast of** the latest research and methods in crisis management so that you are always prepared.

Crisis management relies on a combination of anticipation, skill, effective communication and empathy. With the right training and a patient-centred approach, nurses can effectively manage even the most critical situations and ensure the patient's safety and well-being.

De-escalation strategies

In the dynamic and often unpredictable world of acute medicine, nurses can be faced with situations where patients, or sometimes their relatives, become agitated, anxious or aggressive. At such times, the nurse's ability to de-escalate the situation is crucial, not only to guarantee everyone's safety, but also to ensure that the patient is properly cared for. De-escalation strategies are proven techniques that can help reduce tension and prevent potentially dangerous situations.

- Active listening :
    - **Put yourself at the patient's level:** Face them, make eye contact and show an interest in what they are saying.
    - **Verbal reflection:** Repeating the patient's concerns to show them that they are being heard.
- Non-verbal communication :
    - **Open posture:** Avoid crossing your arms or showing signs of aggression.
    - **Personal space:** Respect the patient's space while guaranteeing their safety and yours.
- Stay calm and in control:
    - **Voice regulation:** Speak in a calm, soothing voice, avoiding shouting or raising your voice.
    - **Breathe in:** Take deep breaths to stay centred and calm.

- Validating feelings :
    - **Acknowledge emotions:** Even if you don't agree with the reasons for the agitation, acknowledge and validate the patient's feelings.

- Establish clear limits:
  - **Explain expectations:** Inform the patient of the expected behaviours and the consequences if they do not comply.
- Choice and autonomy :
  - **Offer options: Wherever possible,** give the patient a sense of control by offering choices.
- Disengagement :
  - **Strategic   withdrawal:** If the situation does not improve, it may be necessary to temporarily leave the area until the patient calms down.
- Call for reinforcements:
  - **Seek help from other team   members:** If necessary, ask other members of staff to help you or consider calling security.
- Training and preparation :
  - **Regular   training:** Make sure you are up to date with de-escalation training and familiar with the facility's protocols.
- Post-incident :
- **Debriefing:** Discuss the incident with the team to identify the lessons to be learned.
- **Support:** Seek emotional support if you need it, whether from colleagues, supervisors or professionals.

The key to successful de-escalation lies in anticipation, effective communication and compassion. By adopting a patient-centred approach and using these strategies, nurses can successfully navigate tense situations, ensuring the safety and well-being of all involved.

Dealing with violence and aggression

Violence and aggression in healthcare, particularly in acute medicine, are a growing concern. Faced with pain, fear or confusion, some patients may react violently. This can also be exacerbated by mental disorders or substance abuse. For nurses, managing these situations is essential to guarantee their safety, that of the team and that of the patient.

- Early recognition :
  - **Signs of threat:** Learn to spot the first signs of agitation, such as a clenched jaw, clenched fist or aggressive posture.
  - **Triggering factors:** Identify the elements that can exacerbate the situation, such as a crowded room or unmet expectations.
- Creating a safe environment:
  - **Layout:** Organise the space to allow easy exit.
  - **Emergency protocols:** Having an alert system to quickly inform colleagues and security of a potentially dangerous situation.
- De-escalation techniques :
  - **Non-confrontational approach:** Adopt an open stance, avoid direct eye contact and use a low, calm tone of voice.
  - **Empathy:** Try to understand the patient's point of view and show empathy for their feelings.
- Maintain distance and barriers :
  - **Personal space:** Keep a safe distance from the agitated patient.
  - **Barriers:** Use items such as a desk or table as a barrier between you and the patient if necessary.

Physical intervention :

Training: Nurses must be trained in non-harmful physical intervention techniques to contain an aggressive patient as a last resort.

The importance of teamwork: Working in coordination with other members of staff to ensure a safe intervention.

Medical support :

Psychiatric consultation: In some cases, a psychiatric assessment may be necessary.

Medication: The administration of sedative drugs may be considered with the agreement of a doctor.

Post-incident :

Debriefing: It is crucial to review the incident with the team to identify possible improvements.

Psychological support: Following a traumatic event, nurses may need to talk and receive support.

Continuing education :

Workshops and simulations: Take part in regular training courses to keep abreast of best practice in violence management.

Prevention :

Patient engagement: Establishing a trusting relationship with patients from the outset can help prevent escalation.

Hospital policies: Ensuring that hospital policies are clear, communicated and implemented.

The key to effective management of violence and aggression lies in preparation, training and a patient-centred approach. By understanding the needs and concerns of the patient and being equipped with the appropriate tools, nurses can successfully navigate these difficult situations while ensuring the safety and well-being of all.

Chapter 16.
THE IMPORTANCE OF DOCUMENTATION

Basic principles of documentation in acute medicine

In acute medicine, where seconds can count and situations change rapidly, accurate and timely documentation is essential. Comprehensive documentation not only ensures effective communication between members of the healthcare team, but also plays a crucial role in continuity of care, legal liability, billing, and quality research and improvement.

- Accuracy and Precision:
  - **Specific details:** Record specific information such as drug dosages, patient reactions or details of a procedure.
  - **Avoid generalities:** Instead of "the patient is fine", opt for "the patient is stable with vital signs within normal limits".
- News :
  - **Real-time documentation: Wherever** possible, document during or immediately after an event or intervention.
  - **Time stamping:** Make sure that each entry is clearly dated and timed.
- Consistency :
  - **Standardised terminology:** Use accepted medical terms and avoid non-standardised abbreviations.
  - **Constant format:** Follow your institution's established standards for formatting and structure.

Completeness :

Full picture: Documentation should reflect a holistic picture of the patient, including history, assessments, interventions and plans.

Avoiding gaps: If something is not documented, it is often assumed not to have happened.

Objectivity :

Be neutral: Record the facts as they are, without adding your own opinion or interpretation.

Direct quotes : If the patient or a family member makes a significant statement, document it in inverted commas.

Confidentiality :

Protect information: Make sure that all documented information is secure and only accessible to those who have the right to see it.

Comply with laws and regulations: Comply with all privacy laws, such as GDPR in Europe or HIPAA in the US.

Revisions and Corrections :

Never erase: If a correction is required, follow the appropriate procedures, usually by drawing a single line through the error and adding the correction.

Sign each entry: Make sure that each entry, correction or addition is accompanied by your initials or signature.

Communication :

Facilitate the transfer of care: Your documentation should enable any healthcare professional to quickly understand the patient's condition and the care they have received.

Refer to other notes: If another specialty (such as cardiology) has been consulted, mention this and refer to their notes for an overview.

Use :

Electronic medical   records: Learn how to use and master your institution's EMR systems for fast, efficient documentation.

Ongoing training: Technology and documentation procedures evolve. Make sure you keep abreast of best practice.

Documentation in acute medicine, although demanding, is a cornerstone of care delivery. It ensures that every patient receives high-quality care based on the most up-to-date and comprehensive information available.

Electronic files and technologies

At the dawn of the digital revolution, the medical world underwent a drastic metamorphosis, transforming itself from a system based on paper records to an environment largely dominated by electronic technologies. This transition, although sometimes complicated, has considerably improved the quality of care, patient safety and collaboration between healthcare professionals. In this context, electronic medical records (EMRs) and other related technologies are playing a predominant role, especially in acute medicine, where time is often a critical factor.

Electronic Medical   Records (EMR) :

Benefits: They guarantee rapid access to comprehensive patient information, promote continuity of care and reduce medical errors.

Integration: The EMR can be interconnected with other hospital systems, such as pharmacies, laboratories or radiology, enabling a continuous flow of information.

Security and confidentiality: Modern systems are equipped with robust security measures to protect patient data.

Telemedicine :

Remote consultations: This enables medical care to be provided via video platforms, which are essential for patients in remote areas.

Remote monitoring: Patients can be monitored remotely using devices that transmit data in real time to healthcare professionals.

Monitoring and warning systems :

Vital signs monitors: These connected devices can alert care staff to anomalies or critical changes in a patient's condition.

Predictive algorithm: Some EMRs use algorithms to predict potential risks to the patient, such as the risk of sepsis or other complications.

Interoperability :

Improved collaboration: EMRs can often communicate between different establishments or specialities, facilitating the transfer of information and responsibilities.

Patient access: Patients can often access their own records, which helps them to be more involved in their care.

Portable technology :

Wearable devices: Many devices, such as smartwatches or wristbands, can now track various health parameters and transmit this information to healthcare professionals.

Mobile applications: There are many applications designed to help you manage illnesses, monitor vital signs or even take medication.

- Training and adaptation :
  - **Ongoing development:** With technology changing so rapidly, ongoing training is essential to ensure safe and effective use.
  - **Ethical and regulatory challenges:** The speed of technological innovation means that regulation and ethics must constantly adapt to protect patients and their data.

At the intersection of technology and medicine, electronic records and related technologies have revolutionised the way care is delivered, particularly in acute situations. Adopting and adapting to these tools is essential for any healthcare professional aspiring to provide the best possible care in the modern world.

Legal aspects and implications documentation

Medical documentation is more than just an administrative formality: it embodies the chronology of the care provided, guarantees patient quality and safety, and has an indisputable legal aspect. In acute medicine, where decisions are often taken in a hurry, accurate and comprehensive documentation is all the more crucial. Omission, inaccuracy or negligence in documentation can have serious legal consequences for healthcare professionals.

- Legal importance of documentation :
  - **Evidence of care provided:** Medical records serve as objective evidence of the care provided, the decisions made and the information shared with the patient.

Professional liability: Inadequate documentation can lead to accusations of negligence or professional misconduct.

Informed consent :

Documenting the process: It is crucial to document that the patient has been properly informed of the risks, benefits and alternatives of a treatment or procedure, and that they have given their informed consent.

Protection against litigation: Appropriate documentation of consent can protect the healthcare professional in the event of accusations of having carried out a treatment or intervention without the patient's consent.

Confidentiality and data protection :

Confidentiality regulations: Healthcare professionals are required by law to protect patients' medical information. Breaches of confidentiality may result in criminal and civil penalties.

Transferring and sharing information: Documentation must be shared securely, particularly when communicating between different establishments or specialities.

Withholding and destruction of files :

Retention period: Local or national laws generally impose a minimum period for which medical records must be kept.

Secure destruction: When records are destroyed, this must be done in such a way as to protect patient confidentiality and privacy.

Patient access to records :

Right of access: In many countries, patients have the right to access their medical records and request copies.

- **Corrections and amendments :** Patients may often request that errors or omissions in their records be corrected. The way in which these corrections are made and documented is important.

- Training and responsibility :

  - **Continuing education:** Healthcare professionals must be regularly trained in the legal requirements for documentation to ensure compliance.

  - **Audit and review:** Establishments can carry out regular audits of documentation to ensure that standards are being met and to identify areas for improvement.

Documentation reflects the professional integrity of a healthcare provider. It is the guarantor of the quality of care, a source of information for the patient and legal protection for the professional. In acute medicine, where every decision can have vital consequences, it is imperative that every detail is understood, analysed and respected.

Chapter 17.
SPECIFIC PROCEDURES
AND THEIR MANAGEMENT

Insertion of probes and catheters

Inserting catheters is an essential skill for nurses working in acute medicine. These devices are commonly used to administer medication, monitor organ function or drain body fluids. Each type has its own set of guidelines, and their use requires technical precision and constant attention to hygiene to avoid complications.

Common types of probes and catheters :

Urinary catheters: Used to drain the bladder, they can be temporary or permanent.

Central venous catheters: inserted into a large vein, usually in the neck, chest or groin, to administer medication or monitor haemodynamics.

Peripheral venous catheters: Used to administer fluids and medicines via the veins in the arms.

Gastric tubes: used to administer food or medication or to drain gastric contents.

Intubation probes: inserted into the trachea in resuscitation situations to provide an airway or administer oxygen.

Integration techniques :

Preparing the patient: The patient needs to be reassured, the procedure explained and consent obtained.

- **Asepsis:** Sterility is essential to avoid infection. Use of sterile gloves, sterile drapes and antiseptics.
- **Insertion itself:** Varies according to the type of catheter. A precise technique is required to guarantee safety.

Maintenance and surveillance :
- **Regular checks:** You need to ensure that the catheter or catheter catheter is always correctly positioned and that there are no signs of infection.
- **Cleaning:** Hygiene around the insertion site must be maintained.
- **Check operation:** Ensure good circulation or drainage, avoid obstructions.

Potential complications :
- **Infections :** An infection may develop around the insertion site or spread throughout the body.
- **Obstruction:** A catheter or probe may become blocked.
- **Trauma:** Incorrect insertion can damage an organ or blood vessel.

Removal of devices :
- **Procedure:** Removal must be carried out with care to avoid trauma.
- **Post-removal monitoring:** Monitor the patient for any signs of complications after removal.

Training and skills :
- **Apprenticeship:** Nurses must be trained and certified to insert these devices.
- **Updates:** As techniques and equipment evolve, skills need to be regularly updated.

Inserting catheters is a common but delicate procedure in acute medicine. Compliance with protocols, impeccable technique and careful monitoring are essential to guarantee patient safety.

Withdrawals and emergency laboratory tests

Taking samples and interpreting laboratory tests are at the heart of patient care in medical emergencies. These analyses offer healthcare professionals a valuable window on the patient's physiological state, guiding diagnosis, treatment and follow-up. For nurses in acute medicine, mastery of this aspect is crucial.

- Importance of samples in acute medicine :
    - **Rapid diagnosis:** To identify the underlying cause of a medical problem.
    - **Progress monitoring:** Assessing the progression of a disease or the effectiveness of a treatment.
    - **Therapeutic decisions:** Adjust treatments according to the results obtained.
- Common types of sampling :
    - **Blood:** haemogram, biochemistry, blood gas, cardiac markers, etc.
    - **Urine:** Standard urine analysis, toxicology test.
    - **Cerebrospinal fluid:** In cases of suspected meningitis or other neurological disorders.
    - **Cultures:** To detect bacterial, viral or fungal infections.
- Sampling techniques :
    - **Site selection:** Choice of vein or suitable body region.

- **Preparing the patient:** Reassuring the patient and obtaining their consent.
- **Aseptic technique:** To prevent contamination or infection.

Emergency laboratory tests :

- **Biochemistry:** renal and liver function, electrolytes, glucose, etc.
- **Haematology:** blood count, coagulation time.
- **Microbiology:** Cultures, antibiogram.
- **Toxicology:** Detection of drugs or toxins in blood or urine.
- **Immunology:** antibody tests, inflammation markers.

Interpretation of results :

- **Normal versus pathological values:** Knowledge of normal ranges and their clinical implications.
- **Clinical correlation:** Relating results to the patient's clinical condition.
- **Anomaly management:** Identify results requiring immediate action.

Communication with the laboratory :

- **Sample transmission:** Ensure that samples are correctly labelled and sent promptly.
- **Exchange of information:** In the event of abnormal or unexpected results, discuss the matter with the technicians or biologists to clarify the results.

Role of the nurse :

- **Accurate sampling:** Ensure the quality of the sample to avoid false negatives or false positives.
- **Safety awareness:** Handle samples with care to avoid any risk of contamination.
- **Patient education:** explaining the tests and their implications to the patient and their family.

Laboratory samples and tests are essential tools in the management of medical emergencies. For nurses, a good command of this aspect guarantees better quality of care, rapid identification of problems and more effective intervention.

Suture techniques and wound care

The ability to suture and care for wounds correctly is an invaluable skill for any nurse working in acute medicine. Whether it's a laceration from an accident or a surgical incision, effective wound management is essential to prevent infection, ensure optimal healing and minimise scarring.

Introduction to wounds :
- **Types of wounds:** Cuts, abrasions, avulsions, bites, burns.
- **Initial assessment:** Depth, length, contamination, presence of foreign bodies.

Preparing the wound :
- **Cleaning:** Use antiseptic solutions to remove contaminants.
- **Local anaesthetic:** Lidocaine or other agents to anaesthetise the area.
- **Removing foreign bodies:** Carefully to avoid aggravating the wound.

Suturing techniques :
- **Simple sutures: The** most common technique for bringing the edges of a wound together.
- **Matra sutures:** Used for deep wounds or to reduce tension.
- **Overlock sutures:** For long linear wounds.

131

- **Intradermal sutures:** When you want to minimise the visible scar.
- **Staples:** For quick fastening, generally on the scalp or trunk.
- **Skin glue:** For small superficial wounds.

Choice of suture :

- **Absorbable vs non-absorbable t h r e a d :** Depending on the site and type of wound.
- **Wire gauge:** Depends on the thinness and tension of the wound.

Post-suture care :

- **Wound protection:** Use of sterile dressings to avoid contamination.
- Monitoring for signs of infection: redness, heat, pain, oozing.
- **Advice for the patient:** Keep the wound clean, avoid excessive movement and observe any complications.

Removal of sutures :

- **Timing:** Depends on the type of suture and the location of the wound.
- **Technique:** Gentle removal to avoid damaging the healed skin.

Complications and their management :

- **Infections :** Prevented by proper cleaning and treated with antibiotics.
- **Hypertrophic or keloid scarring:** Steroid injections, surgery or laser therapy.
- **Disunion:** Re-suturing or other interventions to promote healing.

Role of the nurse :

- **Patient education:** Explanation of wound care, signs of infection, when and how to return for suture removal.
- **Technical skills:** Mastery of suturing techniques for optimal care.

Communication: Ensuring that the patient feels comfortable and informed at every stage.

The ability to suture and heal wounds is an essential part of acute medicine. As well as ensuring optimal healing, effective wound management can greatly improve patient comfort and overall satisfaction. For nurses, this means constantly updating their skills and staying at the cutting edge of best practice.

Chapter 18.
PAIN MANAGEMENT

Pain assessment

Pain, often described as the 'fifth vital constant', is a complex and multifactorial element of the human experience. In acute medicine, rapid and accurate assessment of pain is crucial not only for patient comfort, but also for diagnosing, treating and monitoring the progress of many conditions. The global approach to pain takes into account the physiological, emotional and contextual dimensions, enabling more comprehensive and individualised management.

- Introduction to pain :
  - **Definition:** Unpleasant sensation associated with actual or potential tissue damage.
  - **Types :** Acute vs chronic, nociceptive vs neuropathic.
  - **Mechanisms:** Transduction, transmission, modulation and perception.
- Assessment scales :
  - **Visual analogue (VAS):** The patient situates his or her pain on a graduated line.
  - **Numeric:** From 0 (no pain) to 10 (most intense pain imaginable).
  - **Scales for specific populations:** children, the elderly, non-communicative patients.
- Overall assessment :
  - **Location:** Where is the pain?
  - **Intensity:** How intense is it?
  - **Quality:** Is it throbbing, burning, pulsating?

    Duration and evolution: For how long? Is it constant or intermittent?

    Triggering and alleviating factors: What makes the pain worse or better?

    Associated symptoms: Nausea, shortness of breath, sweating.

Pain and emotion :

    Psychological impact: Pain can be exacerbated by stress, anxiety and depression.

    Mood assessment: How is the patient feeling? Does the pain affect their mood?

The importance of regular assessment :

    Follow-up: To ensure that interventions are effective.

    Prevention: Anticipating and treating pain before it becomes intolerable.

Specific challenges :

    Non-communicative patients: Use of behavioural scales.

    Cultural beliefs: Respecting and understanding patients' perspectives on pain.

Role   of the nurse :

    First line: It is often the nurse who first assesses the patient's pain.

    Patient education: Helping patients to understand their pain and the proposed treatments.

    Collaboration: Working with the care team to ensure optimum care.

Assessing pain is an essential skill for all healthcare professionals, and particularly for nurses in acute medicine. It is often the main and most worrying symptom for the patient. A complete, regular and individualised assessment enables more effective and humane management, reducing patient suffering and speeding up recovery.

Medicines and techniques
non-pharmacological

The treatment of pain and other symptoms in acute medicine is not limited to the administration of drugs. Holistic management incorporates non-pharmacological interventions which, combined with appropriate drug therapy, can offer patients a significant improvement in their comfort and well-being.

Medicines in acute medicine :

- **Analgesics: From** acetaminophen to opioids, these drugs target various pain pathways.
- **Anti-inflammatories:** Commonly used to treat pain associated with inflammation.
- **Sedatives and anxiolytics:** Useful for managing agitation, anxiety or sleep disorders.
- **Antispasmodics:** For muscular pain or cramps.
- **Topical:** Creams, gels or patches applied directly to the painful area.

Non-pharmacological techniques :

- **Heat therapy:** The use of heat or cold can help relieve pain and inflammation.
- **Transcutaneous electrical s t i m u l a t i o n (TENS):** Uses small electrical impulses to reduce the perception of pain.
- **Massage:** Can improve circulation, reduce muscle tension and induce relaxation.
- **Mobilisation and physiotherapy:** Helps strengthen muscles, improve mobility and reduce pain.
- **Relaxation therapies:** deep breathing techniques, meditation or visualisation.
- **Biofeedback:** Learning to control certain bodily functions to help manage pain.

Distraction: Using music, reading or games to divert attention from the pain.

Complementary approaches :

Acupuncture: Inserting fine needles into specific points on the body can help relieve pain.

Aromatherapy: Use of essential oils to induce relaxation and well-being.

Cognitive-behavioural therapies: Techniques to modify the negative thoughts and behaviours associated with pain.

Patient involvement :

Education: helping patients to understand their treatment options and their effectiveness.

Self-management: Encouraging patients to take an active role in managing their pain.

Evaluation and monitoring :

Ongoing evaluation: Ensuring that interventions are effective and adjusting the treatment plan accordingly.

Patient feedback: Patient feedback is essential for assessing the effectiveness of interventions.

The combination of drugs and non-pharmacological techniques allows more comprehensive and individualised management of pain and other symptoms in acute medicine. The multi-dimensional approach is not only more effective, but also respects the wish of many patients to use less invasive and more natural methods to complement traditional drug treatments.

Pain management in specific populations (children, the elderly)

Pain management in acute medicine is a challenge, but when it comes to specific populations such as children and the elderly, this challenge is accentuated. These groups have unique needs, responses and vulnerabilities, and require a tailored and sensitive approach.

1. Pain in children :
a. Recognition and assessment :
- The communication barrier: Very young children cannot adequately express their pain. Using age-appropriate pain scales, such as the FLACC pain scale or the face scale, can help.
- Observe behaviour: Crying, agitation or withdrawal can be indicators of pain.

b. Pharmacological approaches :
- Dosage adapted to weight and age.
- Preference for oral or topical forms, if possible.

c. Non-pharmacological interventions :
- Distraction techniques: toys, stories, music.
- Play therapy to understand and manage pain.
- Parental support: The comfort and presence of parents can reduce anxiety and pain.

2. Pain in the elderly :
a. Recognition and assessment :
- Communication: Cognitive problems can make it difficult to express pain. Appropriate assessment scales, such as the pain scale for non-communicative dementia, can be useful.
- Polypathology: Elderly people may suffer from several pathologies at the same time, which complicates pain assessment.

b. Pharmacological approaches :
  Caution with opioids: Increased risk of side effects such as sedation or constipation.
  Avoid drugs with anticholinergic potential.
  Monitor drug interactions due to polypathology.
c. Non-pharmacological interventions :
  Physical therapies: physiotherapy, gentle massages.
  Cognitive therapies: to manage stress and chronic pain.
  Environment: A comfortable bed, good light and a pleasant temperature can improve comfort.

3. Education and communication :
Whether the patient is a child or an elderly person, educating family members is crucial. Helping them to understand the nature of pain, treatment options and means of support can considerably improve the quality of care.

Although pain management is a fundamental part of acute medicine for all patients, particular attention needs to be paid to specific populations. A patient-centred approach, incorporating both pharmacological and non-pharmacological interventions, is essential to provide appropriate and effective care.

Chapter 19.
THE ROLE OF THE NURSE
IN PREVENTION MEDICAL ERRORS

Common errors in acute medicine

Acute medicine, with its fast pace and emergency situations, is inevitably a breeding ground for errors. These errors can result from a variety of factors, including fatigue, time pressure, faulty systems and poor communication. Understanding these errors is the first step in preventing them.

1. Diagnostic errors :
Acute medicine often requires rapid decisions based on limited information. This can lead to :

- **Misinterpretation of symptoms:** Some symptoms may be wrongly attributed to less serious conditions.
- **Ignoring an essential medical history:** Failing to consider an important medical history can lead to a misdiagnosis.
- **Over-reliance on diagnostic tests:** Tests should not replace clinical assessment.

2. Medication errors :
Medication errors are common in acute medicine because of the complexity and speed of care. They can include :

- **Incorrect doses:** Administering too high or too low a dose.
- **Drug interactions:** Do not take into account any other medicines the patient is already taking.
- **Administration to the wrong patient:** Especially in very busy wards.

3. Communication errors :
Clear communication is essential, but often compromised in stressful environments.

   Care transitions: Errors often occur when patients are transferred from one department to another or from one team to another.

   Non-documentation: Failure to document essential information or to read the patient's notes carefully.

4. Errors relating to equipment and technology :

   Incorrect use of equipment: For example, a defibrillator used incorrectly during resuscitation.

   Technological faults: such as a surveillance monitor that is not working properly.

5. Errors in managing time and priorities :
In an environment where everything seems urgent, it's easy to :

   Neglecting unstable vital signs: Focusing too much on an apparent injury or condition to the detriment of an underlying problem.

   Delaying care for critically ill patients: Sometimes caused by overcrowded emergency rooms.

6. Ignoring the importance of team well-being :
Fatigue, stress and burnout can contribute to errors. Failure to pay attention to the mental and physical health of the medical team can have dramatic consequences.

Recognising common errors in acute medicine is essential to preventing them. Ongoing training, the application of standardised protocols, clear communication, appropriate use of technology and support for the medical team are all approaches that can reduce these errors and ensure the best quality of care for patients.

Safety protocols and checklists

Acute medicine is an area where decisions often have to be taken quickly and under pressure. In this environment, safety protocols and checklists play an essential role in ensuring that every patient receives safe and effective care. These tools are designed to minimise errors, standardise care and provide a solid basis for real-time decision-making.

1. The importance of protocols :
Protocols provide a framework for the management of patients in emergency situations. They provide clear, step-by-step guidelines, based on scientific evidence, for treating a variety of conditions and emergency situations.

2. The value of checklists :
Unlike protocols, which can be more detailed, checklists offer a series of quick points to check. They are particularly useful for ensuring that no steps are forgotten during specific procedures.

3. Common examples of protocols and checklists :
- **Cardiopulmonary resuscitation (CPR):** A standardised protocol for the management of cardiac arrest.
- **Stroke management:** A protocol for the rapid administration of thrombolytic therapy.
- **Intubation checklist:** A checklist of the steps and equipment needed to intubate a patient safely.
- **Transfusion checklist:** To ensure safety when transfusing blood or blood products.

4. Implementation and training :
For these tools to be effective, they must be well designed, widely accessible and regularly updated. In addition, staff

must be trained in their use and understand their importance.

5. Review and continuous improvement :
The effectiveness of protocols and checklists must be regularly evaluated. Feedback from staff, incidents and new medical discoveries can all lead to revisions.

6. Integration with :
With the advent of technology in medicine, many protocols and checklists are now integrated into electronic systems. This can help with speed and accuracy, but it is still essential that staff understand the basis of each step.

In acute medicine, where every second counts, safety protocols and checklists are invaluable. They ensure that the care provided is consistent, based on the best available evidence and geared towards patient safety. Their successful integration requires training, commitment and a willingness to consistently adhere to the highest standards of medical care.

Communication and feedback within the team

The rapid and unpredictable dynamics of acute medicine require clear, concise and effective communication between members of the medical team. Furthermore, constructive and timely feedback is essential for the continuous improvement of skills and processes. The synergy between good communication and effective feedback can mean the difference between life and death in many situations.

1. The importance of clear communication :
In acute medicine, information must be transmitted quickly and unambiguously. Whether it's resuscitation, emergency surgery or complex medical management, every member of the team needs to understand their task, the patient's expectations and objectives.

2. Communication tools and techniques :
  SBAR (Situation, Background, Assessment, Recommendation): A structured method for communicating critical information.

  Briefings and debriefings: Short but essential meetings before and after procedures or emergency situations to make sure everyone is on the same wavelength.

  Verbal and non-verbal signals: It's crucial to be aware of your own non-verbal communication and that of others.

3. Feedback: a tool for growth :
Feedback should not be seen as criticism, but as an opportunity to learn and improve. It should be :
  Opportunistic: Given as soon as possible after observation.

  Specific: Focus on specific actions or behaviours.

  Constructive: Propose solutions or alternatives.

  Caring: Coming from a place of support and encouragement.

4. Overcoming barriers to communication :
  Hierarchy: Encouraging a culture where everyone, whatever their level or role, feels free to speak up and express their concerns.

  Cultural and linguistic differences: Provide training and resources to help staff communicate effectively despite language or cultural barriers.

5. The value of the simulation :
Simulation training enables teams to practise communicating effectively in stressful situations, without risk to patients. It can also help identify areas for improvement in team communication.

Communication and feedback are essential to patient safety and team effectiveness in acute medicine. Creating a culture where communication is valued, feedback is given and received in a spirit of growth, and barriers to effective communication are actively identified and overcome, can improve patient outcomes and strengthen team cohesion and satisfaction.

Chapter 20.
PALLIATIVE APPROACH
IN ACUTE MEDICINE

Understanding palliative medicine

Palliative medicine is a medical speciality that focuses on the prevention and relief of suffering, and on improving the quality of life of patients facing serious and life-threatening illnesses. It focuses on the whole person, integrating the physical, emotional, social and spiritual dimensions of care.

1. What is palliative medicine?
Palliative medicine is an approach that improves the quality of life of patients (and their families) faced with problems related to life-threatening illnesses, through the prevention and relief of suffering, and the comprehensive and careful assessment of pain and other physical, psychological and spiritual symptoms.

2. The basic principles :
   Global approach: Care goes beyond the treatment of physical pain to encompass emotional, psychological and spiritual needs.
   Interdisciplinarity: The palliative care team generally includes doctors, nurses, social workers, therapists and spiritual advisers working together.
   Respecting the patient's wishes: Patients and their families are at the heart of decisions about their care.

3. Palliative medicine is not synonymous with the end of life:
Although it may be associated with end-of-life care, palliative medicine can be introduced at any stage of a serious illness, alongside other curative treatments.

4. Managing pain and other symptoms :
Palliative medicine aims to effectively manage pain and other troublesome symptoms, whether physical (nausea, shortness of breath), emotional (anxiety, depression) or spiritual.

5. Emotional and spiritual support :
Recognising that serious illness and death can lead to existential crises, palliative care seeks to offer appropriate emotional and spiritual support.

6. Discussion on the end of life :
Palliative medicine professionals help patients and their families to understand the illness, set goals of care and make informed decisions about future treatment.

7. Palliative care at home :
The aim is often to enable the patient to remain at home, in familiar surroundings, while receiving the necessary care and support.

8. The difference between palliative care and end-of-life care :
While all end-of-life care is palliative in nature, not all palliative care is necessarily provided at the end of life.

Palliative medicine strives to see the whole person, recognising that suffering can manifest itself in many different ways. It aims to ensure quality of life, however long it may be, by placing the patient and those close to him or her at the centre of its concerns.

Symptom management at the end of life

The end of life is a delicate period, often accompanied by a variety of symptoms that require careful management.

These symptoms may be physical, emotional, psychological or spiritual. Managing these symptoms is at the heart of palliative medicine, which aims to ensure patient comfort while respecting their wishes and needs.

1. Pain :
   - **Assessment:** The first step is to understand the cause, type, intensity and frequency of the pain.
   - **Treatments:** These may include analgesics, anti-inflammatories, nerve blocks and non-medicinal therapies such as massage therapy or acupuncture.
2. Shortness of breath :
   - **Common causes:** Heart problems, pneumonia, pleural or tumour effusion.
   - **Management:** Oxygen, bronchodilator drugs, sitting up and ventilators can help.
3. Nausea and vomiting :
   - **Causes:** Medication, constipation, intestinal obstruction or brain metastases.
   - **Treatments :** Anti-emetic medication, dietary adjustments and complementary therapies such as ginger or acupressure.
4. Agitation and delirium :
   - **Identification of causes:** medication, infection, electrolyte imbalance, or disease progression.
   - **Management:** Medication re-evaluation, palliative sedation, calm environment, presence of relatives.
5. Insomnia :
   - **Causes:** Pain, medication, anxiety or depression.
   - **Treatments :** Sedatives, bedtime rituals, relaxation therapies.
6. Constipation :
   - **Causes:** Immobility, medication such as opioids, dehydration.
   - **Management:** Laxatives, high-fibre diet, hydration.

7. Psychological and emotional symptoms :

   Recognition: Feelings of sadness, anxiety, anger, fear or isolation.

   Interventions: counselling, therapy, support groups, medication, relaxation techniques.

8. Spiritual symptoms :

   Manifestations: Questions about the meaning of life, reconciliation, forgiveness or fear of death.

   Accompaniment: Spiritual talks, religious rites, meditation, accompaniment by a chaplain or spiritual adviser.

Managing symptoms at the end of life requires a multi-dimensional approach that respects the unique needs of each patient. While some symptoms can be treated with medical interventions, others may require a more holistic approach, integrating psychological, emotional and spiritual aspects. The key is open communication between the patient, the family and the medical team, enabling individualised care that aims to provide comfort and dignity in this crucial phase of life.

Communication with patients and families

Communication is at the heart of medical practice. For nurses in acute medicine, it is all the more crucial, as it often takes place at times of crisis, uncertainty and vulnerability for patients and their families. The way in which information is conveyed can greatly influence the perception of care, patient satisfaction and even clinical outcomes.

1. Making contact :

   First impressions: A smile, eye contact and a handshake can build trust.

Introduce yourself: state your name and your role to clarify your position in the care team.
2. Active listening :
   Show interest: Give the patient or family your undivided attention, without interruption.
   Body language: Positioning yourself in front of the patient, making eye contact and nodding show your involvement.
3. Ask open-ended questions :
   Encourage patients to share their concerns and symptoms by asking questions such as "Tell me about your pain" rather than "Are you in pain?".
4. Validate feelings :
   Recognising the patient's or family's emotions, whether fear, anxiety or frustration, is crucial to establishing a relationship of trust.
5. Use understandable language :
   Avoid medical jargon. Adapt your language to the patient's level of understanding.

6. Inform and educate :
   Regular updates: Keep the patient and family informed of progress, test results and treatment plans.
   Educational material: Brochures or videos can help clarify complex concepts.
7. Clarify and repeat :
   Patients under stress may find it difficult to retain information. Repeat key points and check for understanding.
8. Involving families :
   Relatives can provide valuable information, support the patient and help with decision-making.
9. Dealing with bad news :
   Find a quiet place, sit down and be empathetic and direct. Allow time for questions and emotional reactions.

10. Concluding the conversation :
Summarise the key points, confirm the action plan
and thank the patient or family for their time.

Communication is not just a matter of passing on
information. It is the foundation of a therapeutic
relationship, facilitating understanding, trust and
collaboration. For nurses in acute medicine, mastering this
art is essential to ensure optimal patient care and to
support their loved ones at what are often difficult times.

Chapter 21.
SPECIALIST NURSING CARE

Acute cardiological care

When it comes to acute cardiovascular disease, time is precious and every second counts. Nurses play a crucial role in the early recognition, initial management and follow-up of patients with cardiac conditions. Find out how nurses intervene in acute cardiac situations.

1. Recognising an emergency :
The ability to rapidly detect the signs of an acute cardiac event is vital if appropriate treatment is to be instituted.

- **Classic cardiac symptoms:** Chest pain or discomfort, shortness of breath, excessive sweating, nausea or vomiting.
- **Less typical signs:** Particularly in women, diabetics and the elderly, symptoms may include unexplained fatigue, abdominal pain or dizziness.

2. Initial intervention :
The "B.A.S.E." approach (Bilan, Aspirine, Scope, Electrocardiogram) approach is a simple and effective way of remembering the initial steps.

- **Assessment:** Rapidly assess the patient's condition.
- **Aspirin:** Use aspirin to prevent coagulation, unless contraindicated.
- **Scope:** Put the patient on cardiac monitoring.
- **Electrocardiogram (ECG):** An ECG should be performed within the first 10 minutes to identify cardiac abnormalities.

3. Specialist care :
Depending on the heart condition diagnosed, different operations may be required:

- **Acute coronary syndrome (ACS):** Includes myocardial infarction (heart attack) and unstable angina. Treatment is aimed at restoring blood flow to the heart.
- **Acute heart failure: Treatment is** aimed at improving heart function and reducing symptoms such as breathlessness.

4. Commonly used medicines :
Pharmacotherapy is central to the management of cardiac emergencies.

- **Antiplatelet agents:** Aspirin, clopidogrel.
- **Anticoagulants :** Heparin, enoxaparin.
- **Beta-blockers:** Metropolol, atenolol.
- **Nitroglycerine:** To relieve chest pain.

5. Patient education :
Nurses play a central role in educating patients about how to modify risk factors.

- **Smoking cessation:** Supporting and guiding patients towards smoking cessation programmes.
- **Diet:** Encourage a balanced diet, low in salt and saturated fats.
- **Physical activity:** Discuss the gradual resumption of physical activity after the cardiac event.

6. Preparing for the trip :
Referral does not stop when the patient leaves hospital. The nurse must ensure that the patient :

- Understands the importance of taking medication regularly.
- Knows the warning signs of a relapse or worsening.
- Has follow-up appointments with his cardiologist.

Managing cardiac emergencies requires a rapid, coordinated and evidence-based response. Acute nurses are at the forefront of this response, providing critical care, education and support to help patients navigate the complex world of cardiac conditions.

Acute neurological care

The nervous system, a complex network that controls and coordinates all the body's activities, can be subject to a number of disorders. When faced with an acute neurological pathology, rapid and competent intervention is essential. Nurses are often the first to assess, manage and monitor these patients, playing a vital role in their outcome.

1. Recognising symptoms :
Neurological pathologies can manifest themselves in different ways. Knowing how to identify them is crucial.
- **Signs of stroke:** facial paralysis, weakness or numbness on one side of the body, difficulty speaking or understanding.
- **Symptoms of a meningeal haemorrhage :** Sudden, intense headaches, stiff neck, sensitivity to light.

2. Initial assessment :
The first hour following a neurological event is often referred to as the "golden hour", underlining the urgency of treatment.
- **Neurological examination:** Assess brain function, level of consciousness, motor skills, sensitivity, reflexes and signs of engagement.
- **Brain imaging:** A brain scan or MRI is often performed to identify the cause of the incident.

3. Specialist care :
Care depends on the underlying pathology.
- **Ischaemic stroke:** Thrombolysis to dissolve the clot responsible for the ischaemia, if the patient is eligible.

Cerebral haemorrhage: Close monitoring, blood pressure control, possible surgery to relieve pressure.

4. Commonly used drugs :

Antithrombotics: To prevent the formation of blood clots.

Antihypertensives: To manage blood pressure.

Anticonvulsants : In the event of epileptic seizures.

5. Continuous monitoring :

Vital signs: Regular monitoring to detect changes.

Glasgow scale: To assess the level of consciousness.

6. Education and support :

Recognising warning signs: Educating patients and their families to recognise the warning signs of a neurological problem.

Rehabilitation: Neurological sequelae may require motor rehabilitation, speech therapy or occupational therapy.

7. Preparing for the trip :

Re-education and rehabilitation are often necessary after an acute neurological event. Nurses play a central role in :

Ensure that the patient receives the appropriate medication.

Coordinating care with rehabilitation professionals.

Regular follow-up with the neurologist.

The challenges posed by acute neurological conditions require specialised, multidisciplinary care. Thanks to their training and their ability to work closely with a medical team, nurses are essential in ensuring optimal care for these patients, from initial assessment through to rehabilitation.

Acute respiratory care

The respiratory system, dedicated to supplying essential oxygen to our cells and expelling carbon dioxide, can quickly become disrupted. Acute respiratory conditions can be fatal if not treated quickly. Acute care nurses are often on the front line when it comes to intervening, assessing and monitoring patients suffering from such conditions.

1. Understanding the mechanisms :
Each respiratory condition has its own specific features. Understanding them is fundamental to appropriate treatment.

- **Respiratory physiology:** Understanding the basic principles of ventilation, diffusion and perfusion.
- **Interpretation of blood gases:** Assess oxygen saturation, CO_2 levels and acid-base balance.

2. Common symptoms :
Respiratory disorders often manifest as symptoms that require rapid assessment.

- **Dyspnoea:** Difficulty breathing, feeling of suffocation.
- **Cyanosis:** Bluish discolouration of the skin due to low oxygenation.
- **Stridor:** High-pitched respiratory noise indicating upper airway obstruction.

3. Emergency care :
Some situations require immediate intervention.

- **Respiratory arrest: Initiate** assisted ventilation.
- **Pulmonary oedema:** Administration of oxygen, diuretics and sometimes mechanical ventilation.
- **Severe acute asthma:** Administration of bronchodilators, corticosteroids and oxygen.

4. Ventilation techniques :
In severe cases, respiratory assistance may be required.

- **Non-invasive ventilation (NIV):** Supply of oxygen through a mask, without intubation.

Invasive mechanical ventilation: when the patient is intubated and connected to a respirator.

5. Commonly used medicines :

Bronchodilators: To open the airways.

Corticosteroids: To reduce lung inflammation.

Antibiotics: For respiratory infections.

6. Education and support :

Respiratory hygiene education: teaching patients breathing and expectoration techniques.

Infection prevention : Vaccination and barrier measures.

7. Preparing for the trip :

Nurses play an essential role in preventing re-hospitalisation.

Advice on medication compliance.

Education on recognising signs of aggravation.

Coordination with the pulmonologist and respiratory rehabilitation professionals.

Acute respiratory care highlights the delicacy of our respiratory system and the importance of rapid and appropriate intervention. The expertise, observation skills and commitment of nurses in acute medicine are essential to ensuring the best possible care for patients with respiratory problems.

Chapter 22.
MANAGEMENT
ENVIRONMENTAL EMERGENCIES

Hypothermia and hyperthermia

The thermal balance of the human body is essential to the proper functioning of our systems and organs. Any significant variation, whether a fall or a rise in body temperature, can have serious consequences. Acute care nurses must be prepared to identify and deal with these situations quickly.

1. Understanding the mechanisms :
Thermal homeostasis is a complex process involving numerous mechanisms.

- **Thermal regulation:** The role of the hypothalamus, the main regulator of body temperature.
- **External and internal factors:** Influence of the environment, metabolic activity, infections, drugs.

2. Hypothermia: the cold that puts you at risk

- **Causes and risk factors:** Prolonged exposure to cold, immersion in cold water, hypoglycaemia, trauma, certain medical conditions.
- **Symptoms:** Chills, confusion, heart rhythm disturbances, weakness.
- **Management:** Progressive rewarming, monitoring of vital functions, administration of warm fluids, use of warming blankets.
- **Complications:** Cardiac arrest, frostbite, acute renal failure.

3. Hyperthermia: the heat that consumes

- **Causes and risk factors:** Heat waves, intense physical effort, certain drugs, neuroleptic malignant syndromes.
- **Symptoms:** Hot, dry skin, confusion, convulsions, tachycardia.
- **Treatment:** Rapid cooling, hydration, antipyretics, ventilation.
- **Complications:** Dehydration, acute renal failure, coagulation disorders.

4. Routine interventions :

- **Rapid assessment:** Measurement of body temperature, assessment of state of consciousness.
- **Management of dehydration:** Administration of intravenous fluids.
- **Monitoring:** Continuous monitoring of temperature, heart rate and blood pressure.

5. Prevention :

- **Patient education:** Raising awareness of the dangers of extreme temperatures, the importance of protecting yourself from the cold or heat, hydration.
- **Advice for families:** Recognise the signs of hypothermia or hyperthermia, and when to seek medical help.

Hypothermia and hyperthermia, although opposite in nature, are both medical emergencies requiring rapid and specialised care. Acute care nurses play a key role in identifying, treating and preventing these thermal disturbances, thereby guaranteeing the well-being and safety of patients.

Animal bites and stings

Inadvertent encounters with wildlife, whether domestic or wild, can sometimes result in painful and potentially serious injuries. Whether it's dog bites, spider bites or attacks by other animals, acute care nurses are often the first to intervene to assess and treat these injuries.

1. Recognising the different types of injury :
Each animal has a distinct anatomy and behaviour, which is reflected in the type and severity of injuries it can inflict.
   - **Bites:** The consequences of fangs, beaks, etc.
   - **Stings:** Stings, thorns, prickles.
2. Common bites :
   - **Dog bites:** Signs of infection, the importance of rapid assessment, prevention.
   - **Cat bites:** Increased risk of infection, therapeutic approach.
   - **Other domestic and wild animals:** Recognising and treating injuries caused by rodents, snakes and exotic animals.
3. Common injections :
   - **Insects :** Bees, wasps, mosquitoes, fleas, ticks.
   - **Spiders :** Potentially toxic stings and their symptoms, management of complications.
   - **Marine animals:** jellyfish, sea urchins, rays.
4. Initial treatment :
   - **Assessment:** Inspection of the wound, assessment of pain, check on vaccination status (tetanus).
   - **Cleaning and disinfection:** The best way to prevent infection.
   - **Symptomatic treatment:** management of pain, allergic reactions and oedema.
5. Potential complications :
   - **Infections:** symptoms, treatment, prevention.

Allergic reactions: From local reactions to anaphylaxis.

  Toxins and venoms: Antidotes and specific treatments.

6. Prevention :

  Patient education: how to avoid bites and stings, safe behaviour.

  Advice for pet owners: training, vaccinations, responsibilities.

Animal bites and stings can range from simple irritations to medical emergencies. Rapid assessment and appropriate management are essential to minimise complications. Acute care nurses, with their skills and experience, are vital in managing these incidents, ensuring an effective response and reassuring injured patients.

Toxic exposure and poisoning

In the world of acute medicine, toxic poisoning and exposure account for a significant number of admissions. These situations may arise following a domestic accident, deliberate ingestion in a suicidal context or occupational exposure. From the rapid detection of symptoms to the administration of specific treatments, nurses play an essential role in providing care.

1. Recognition of toxic exposure :

  Exposure history: Identify the substance, route of exposure and time elapsed.

  Initial symptoms: The signs generally observed depend on the toxic substance ingested or encountered.

2. Common types of exposure :
- **Medicines:** Intentional or accidental overdose, drug interactions.
- **Household products:** detergents, cleaning agents, insecticides.
- **Industrial products:** Occupational exposure, inhalation of toxic vapours.
- **Plants and fungi:** Recognition and specific symptoms.
- **Illegal substances :** Opiates, stimulants, hallucinogens.

3. Clinical assessment :
- **Triage and initial assessment:** vital signs, neurological status, gastrointestinal symptoms.
- **Diagnostic tests:** blood gases, specific toxic levels, imaging.

4. Therapeutic interventions :
- **Decontamination:** Gastric lavage, administration of activated charcoal, chelation.
- **Support for vital functions:** Ventilation, cardiovascular support drugs, electrolyte corrections.
- **Antidotes:** Specific use depending on the poison, e.g. Naloxone for opiate overdoses.

5. Monitoring and surveillance :
- **Continuous monitoring:** monitoring of vital signs, neurological status, kidney and liver functions.
- **Specialist consultation:** Involvement of a toxicologist or poison control centre.

6. Education and prevention :
- **Advice for the home:** Safe storage of medicines and toxic products.
- **Community information:** risk awareness, workshops, school activities.

7. Psychosocial aspects :
- **Psychiatric assessment:** For voluntary ingestions or self-destructive behaviour.

Support: Encourage discussions with social workers, psychologists or other mental health professionals.

When faced with poisoning or toxic exposure, nurses play a pivotal role. Whether assessing the situation, administering appropriate treatment or supporting the patient and their family, their presence and skills are crucial. The ability to act quickly and effectively in these situations can mean the difference between life and death, underlining the importance of training and preparation in this particular area of acute medicine.

Chapter 23.
MANAGEMENT OF ACUTE PSYCHIATRIC SITUATIONS

Assessment of psychiatric patients

In an acute medical ward, nurses are regularly confronted with patients presenting with psychiatric disorders, whether underlying or acute. Accurate and empathetic assessment of these patients is essential to ensure their safety and well-being, while establishing an appropriate care plan.

1. Initial approach :
   - **A caring attitude:** Establishing a relationship of trust is essential for gathering reliable information and for patient safety.
   - **Safety assessment:** Identify immediate risks, such as aggressiveness or suicidal thoughts.
2. Detailed history :
   - **Reason for consultation:** What is the main reason for the visit or hospitalisation?
   - **Psychiatric history:** previous episodes, treatments, hospitalisations.
3. Assessment of mental state :
   - **General appearance:** Behaviour, clothing, hygiene.
   - **Behaviour:** Agitation, apathy, trembling, unusual postures.
   - **Mood and affect:** Sad, euphoric, flat, labile.
   - **Speeches:** Speed, consistency, relevance.
   - **Thought:** Coherence, content (delusions, hallucinations).
   - **Perception:** auditory, visual, olfactory and tactile hallucinations.
   - Orientation and awareness: place, time, situation.

Memory: short term, long term.

Cognitive skills: Attention, concentration, judgement.

Suicidal or homicidal ideation: presence, plan, means, antecedents.

4. Investigation of past history :

Medical: illnesses, treatments, surgery.

Psychiatric: Previous disorders, hospitalisations, medication.

Social: family and professional situation, lifestyle habits.

5. Physical assessment :

Looking for physical symptoms: Some disorders, such as depression, can be accompanied by physical symptoms such as fatigue or headaches.

Neurological examination: To rule out organic pathologies that may mimic psychiatric disorders.

6. Planning the care plan :

Stabilisation: Ensuring patient safety, treating acute symptoms.

Referral: Depending on severity and diagnosis, psychiatric hospitalisation, specialist consultation or outpatient follow-up.

7. Education and advice :

Information: Explain the patient's condition and proposed treatments.

Resources: Useful contacts, support groups, help structures.

Assessing a psychiatric patient in an acute setting requires both specific clinical skills and the ability to empathise and listen. Nurses are often at the forefront of this assessment, playing a crucial role in detecting disorders, ensuring patient safety and providing appropriate care. It is therefore essential for nurses to be well trained and to have the resources they need to provide the best possible support for these patients at what are often difficult times.

Crisis management linked to disorders mood disorders, psychoses and other

At the heart of acute medical services, nurses are frequently confronted with patients suffering from mood disorders, psychoses or other psychiatric pathologies which can suddenly worsen. Managing these crises is crucial not only for the safety and well-being of the patient, but also for the nursing staff and other patients.

1. Understanding disorders :
   - **Mood disorders:** such as major depression or bipolar disorder, where patients may experience profound sadness, anhedonia or, conversely, excessive euphoria.
   - **Psychoses:** Such as schizophrenia, where patients may experience hallucinations, delusions or social withdrawal.
   - **Anxiety disorders, personality disorders and others:** Each pathology has its own manifestations and associated risks.
2. Initial assessment :
   - **Establishing contact:** Communicate calmly, making eye contact and using the patient's first name.
   - **Assessing the level of agitation:** Identifying signs of aggression or dangerousness.
3. De-escalation techniques :
   - **Active listening:** Validating the patient's feelings without necessarily validating their delusions or hallucinations.
   - **Personal space:** Respecting the patient's personal bubble, while ensuring that there is an accessible exit.
   - **Suggest solutions:** such as a quiet room, medication or a meeting with a specialist.

4. Use of medicines :

- **Anxiolytics or sedatives:** Used to calm a very agitated or aggressive patient.
- **Antipsychotics:** If the patient presents acute psychotic symptoms.
- **Mood stabilisers: In the** event of a manic episode in a bipolar patient.

5. Safety measures :

- **Patient isolation:** In a secure room if necessary, for his/her own safety and that of others.
- **Physical restraint: As a** last resort, with medical authorisation, and always respecting the patient's dignity.

6. In-depth assessment :

- **Past history:** Understand the context of the attack, medication taken, adherence to treatment, etc.
- **Potential triggers:** Life events, substance used, etc.

7. Care plan planning :

- **Specialist referral:** admission to a psychiatric unit, consultation with a psychiatrist or psychologist.
- **Regular monitoring:** To avoid relapses and ensure comprehensive care.

8. Education and awareness :

- **Therapies:** Encourage the patient to take part in therapies, support groups or workshops.
- **Medication:** Explain the importance of adherence to treatment and potential side effects.

When faced with acute psychiatric crises, nurses must act with speed, skill and compassion. The key is to balance the urgency of the situation with respect for the patient's dignity. This requires adequate training, appropriate resources and the ability to work as part of a team. Every crisis is unique, but with the right skills and the right approach, nurses can make a significant difference to the lives of their patients.

Management of suicidal patients

The encounter with a suicidal patient is one of the most delicate and complex challenges that healthcare professionals can face in acute medicine. The potential seriousness and urgent nature of the situation call for immediate, meticulous and compassionate care.

1. Initial assessment :
   - **Establish a relationship of trust:** Adopt a calm, non-judgemental and empathetic approach to encourage patients to express themselves.
   - **Determining risk:** Ask direct questions about suicidal ideation, plans, means and intentions. Try to understand whether there have been previous attempts or a family history.
2. Safety first:
   - **Removal of equipment:** Make sure the patient has no access to potential sharp objects, medicines or other aids.
   - **Continuous monitoring:** High-risk patients may require constant monitoring to ensure their safety.
3. Investigation of triggering factors :
   - **Recent life events:** Loss, break-ups, professional or academic failures, trauma, etc.
   - **Psychopathological conditions:** depression, personality disorders, psychosis, anxiety disorders, addiction, etc.
4. Medication support :
   - **Psychotropic medication:** Certain antidepressants, anxiolytics or antipsychotics may be prescribed, depending on the underlying condition.
   - **Monitoring side-effects:** Some medicines can temporarily increase the risk of suicide, particularly in young people.

5. Interprofessional collaboration :

Psychiatric consultation: A more in-depth assessment by a psychiatrist is often necessary.

Networking: Psychologists, social workers, counsellors, therapists and the family can all play a crucial role in providing care.

6. Drawing up a safety plan :

Avoid isolation: Encourage the patient to remain surrounded by trusted family and friends.

Emergency contact: Make sure the patient has access to emergency numbers or resources in the event of a crisis.

7. Guidance and follow-up :

Hospitalisation: In high-risk cases, hospitalisation in a psychiatric unit may be necessary.

Regular follow-up: The first days and weeks after the attack are crucial. Make sure the patient has close medical and psychological monitoring.

8. Education and prevention :

Avoid alcohol and drugs: These substances can exacerbate suicidal thoughts.

Encourage people to talk: Stress the importance of talking about emotions and thoughts, without judgement or stigmatisation.

Managing a suicidal patient requires a holistic approach, focusing on safety, risk assessment and ongoing support. Each patient is unique, and a deep understanding of their personal and medical challenges is essential. In acute medicine, professionals must be armed with the skills, knowledge and compassion to navigate through these delicate moments, always in the hope of protecting and saving lives.

Chapter 24.
EMERGENCY SURGERY

The role of the nurse
in surgical preparation

Surgical preparation is a crucial stage in ensuring that the operation goes smoothly and minimising post-operative complications. The nurse plays a central role in this process, acting as a link between the patient, the family and the medical-surgical team.

1. Preoperative assessment :

   Data collection: The nurse collects medical history, allergies, current medications, surgical history, and other relevant information to assess surgical risk.

   Physical examination: Although brief, this examination provides vital information about the patient's condition prior to surgery.

2. Patient education :

   Information on the procedure: The nurse explains the nature of the procedure, how it is carried out, the associated risks and the recovery process.

   Mental preparation: The nurse offers emotional support, answers questions and allays the patient's worries.

3. Physical preparation :

   Fasting: The nurse ensures that the patient understands and complies with the instructions concerning fasting before the operation.

   Skin preparation: Depending on the surgery, skin disinfection or shaving may be necessary.

Medication: Administration of preoperative drugs such as antiseptics, prophylactic antibiotics or anxiolytics.

4. Administrative checks :

Informed consent: The nurse ensures that the patient has fully understood the procedure and its risks, and has signed the consent form.

Coordination with the team: The nurse confirms the schedule for the operation, the type of anaesthetic and any other logistical details.

5. Emotional support :

Support: The nurse reassures the patient and their family, offering them a space to express their fears or concerns.

6. Anticipating post-operative needs :

Education: The nurse informs the patient about post-operative care, pain management, mobilisation, nutrition, etc.

Preparation of devices: Ensures that all equipment required for post-operative care (drains, catheters, analgesia pumps, etc.) is ready and functional.

7. Coordination with the surgical team :

Communication: The nurse acts as a link between the patient, the anaesthetist, the surgeon and any other member of the team, ensuring a smooth transition from the patient to the operating theatre.

The surgical preparation nurse is an essential pillar of the surgical process. Their ability to assess, educate, support and coordinate ensures not only that the operation runs smoothly, but also the patient's well-being and safety. This multifunctionality reflects the complexity and richness of the surgical nursing profession.

Immediate post-operative care

After surgery, immediate post-operative care is essential to ensure patients recover quickly, prevent complications and ensure their safety. This care, often administered in the recovery room or intensive care unit, requires continuous attention and monitoring.

1. Vital signs :
    - **Vital signs:** Regular monitoring of blood pressure, pulse, respiration and temperature.
    - **Oxygen saturation:** SpO2 monitoring to detect any postoperative hypoxia.
2. Neurological assessment :
    - **Awareness:** Regular checks on the level of awareness, orientation and ability to respond to simple commands.
    - **Pupillary reflexes:** These are checked to ensure adequate cerebral perfusion and function.
3. Pain management :
    - **Assessment:** The nurse regularly assesses the patient's pain using standardised scales.
    - **Medication:** Administration of prescribed analgesics and adjustment according to pain assessment.
4. Monitoring respiratory function :
    - **Observation:** Monitoring the frequency and depth of breathing, as well as respiratory effort.
    - **Auscultation:** Listening to breath sounds to detect abnormalities such as crackles or sibilants.
5. Monitoring cardiovascular function :
    - **Monitoring:** Continuous monitoring of the electrocardiogram to detect arrhythmias or signs of ischaemia.
    - **Verification** of coloration, temperature and capillary perfusion of the extremities.

6. Monitoring the surgical site :

Inspection: Visual check for bleeding, haematoma or infection.

Drains and catheters: Monitoring the flow and appearance of flows.

7. Monitoring renal function :

Diuresis: Regular measurement of the quantity and appearance of urine.

Urinary catheter: Checking operation and preventing associated infections.

8. Hydration and electrolyte balance :

Administration: Monitoring of intravenous infusions, checking the flow rate and infusion site.

Reports: Keeping up-to-date records of fluids in and out, and anticipating hydration needs.

9. Gastrointestinal assessment :

Nausea and vomiting: Prevention and treatment of postoperative nausea.

Perception of intestinal sounds: Auscultation to assess the return of intestinal motility.

10. Communication :

Reassurance: reassuring patients, informing them of the success of the operation and answering any questions they may have.

Transition: Preparing the patient for transfer to a care unit or their room.

Immediate post-operative care requires expertise, attention and rapid action. Nurses position themselves as first responders, anticipating and managing potential complications, while offering emotional support to the patient who has just undergone an operation. This is a crucial moment when skill, compassion and collaboration combine to ensure the best outcome for the patient.

Management of surgical complications

Surgery, no matter how carefully performed, inevitably entails the risk of complications. These complications may arise during the operation itself, or during the post-operative period. Prompt and effective management of these complications is essential to minimise the after-effects and maximise the patient's chances of making a full recovery.

1. Post-operative haemorrhage :
   - **Recognition:** A sudden drop in blood pressure, tachycardia, pallor and weakness may indicate haemorrhage.
   - **Intervention:** The nurse must immediately alert the surgical team, stop any anticoagulants, administer intravenous fluids and prepare the patient for any investigations or re-operation.
2. Surgical site infection :
   - **Recognition:** Redness, heat, pain, swelling and purulent discharge from the surgical site are typical signs.
   - **Intervention:** Clean the wound, take samples for bacteriological analysis, administer antibiotics as prescribed and monitor closely.

3. Venous thromboembolism :
   - **Recognition:** Pain, swelling and redness of a limb are signs of deep vein thrombosis. A pulmonary embolism may manifest as dyspnoea, chest pain and syncope.
   - **Intervention:** Immobilisation of the patient, administration of anticoagulants, close monitoring and possibly imaging exploration.

4. Post-operative island :
   Recognition: Absence of intestinal sounds, abdominal distension, vomiting and absence of gas or stools.
   Intervention: Maintenance of fasting, gastric aspiration and close monitoring.
5. Dehiscence or evisceration of the wound :
   Recognition: Separation of the edges of the wound, possibly with protrusion of the internal organs.
   Intervention: Cover the wound with a moist sterile dressing, place the patient in a semi-seated position and immediately alert the surgical team.
6. Pulmonary complications :
   Recognition: Dyspnoea, cyanosis, chest pain and reduced or absent breath sounds may indicate pneumothorax, atelectasis or pneumonia.
   Intervention: oxygen therapy, respiratory physiotherapy, antibiotics if necessary and possibly thoracocentesis.
7. Renal complications :
   Recognition: Decreased or absent urine output, swelling, elevated serum creatinine.
   Intervention: Hydration, adjustment of medication, close monitoring and possibly dialysis.
8. Neurological complications :
   Recognition: Changes in consciousness, weakness, paralysis, difficulty speaking.
   Intervention: Regular neurological monitoring, brain scan or MRI, adjustment of medication.

Early recognition and effective management of surgical complications are essential to ensure patient safety. The nurse plays a central role, often being the first to identify a complication. Effective communication with the surgical team, a thorough knowledge of the warning signs and a rapid response can make the difference between a favourable outcome and a tragic one.

Chapter 25.
NURSING CARE
IN A PANDEMIC SITUATION

Pandemic preparedness and response

In the modern world, pandemics can spread rapidly due to population density and the increased mobility of people. Recent history, with the COVID-19 pandemic, is a striking example of this. Pandemic preparedness and response are essential to minimise the impact on public health and the economy.

1. Assessment and monitoring :
    Early recognition: Epidemiological surveillance systems must be put in place to detect new infections or changes in existing disease trends quickly.
    Data collection: Ensure rapid and accurate data collection to understand the nature and spread of the disease.
2. Planning and coordination :
    Contingency planning: Each country must have a detailed contingency plan to deal with a pandemic, including the resources needed, procedures and roles.
    Coordination: Fluid communication between governments, healthcare organisations and the private sector is crucial to a unified and effective response.
3. Medical resources :
    Stockpiles: It is vital to stockpile medicines, vaccines (if available), personal protective equipment and respirators.

Infrastructure : Preparing field hospitals, isolation units and increasing the capacity of existing hospitals.

4. Education and communication :

Public information: Use all available channels to inform the public about symptoms, modes of transmission and preventive measures.

Training healthcare professionals: Ensure that all medical staff are properly trained to recognise, treat and prevent transmission.

5. Public health measures :

Isolation and quarantine: Rapidly isolate infected people and, if necessary, quarantine affected areas.

Social distancing: In the event of rapid transmission, implement social distancing measures, including closing schools and workplaces and cancelling public events.

Travel: Regulate, limit or even prohibit travel to and from the affected areas.

6. Research and development :

Research: Carrying out studies to understand the disease, how it is transmitted and its impact.

Development: Investing in research to develop treatments and vaccines.

7. Psychosocial support :

Mental support: Recognise that pandemics can have a major psychological impact on individuals and set up support systems.

Community: Encouraging acts of solidarity and community mutual aid to overcome the crisis together.

8. Post-pandemic evaluation :

Review: Once the pandemic is under control, carry out a full review of the actions taken to identify areas for improvement.

Preparing for the future: Using lessons learned to strengthen preparedness and response to future pandemics.

Preparing for and responding to a pandemic requires unprecedented coordination at all levels of society. Anticipation, flexibility and solidarity are essential to minimise the impact on health and the economy. While each pandemic presents its own challenges, the fundamental principles of preparedness and response remain constant.

Personal protection and transmission prevention

Personal protection and prevention of transmission are crucial in any healthcare environment, but they become even more essential in acute medicine, where the speed of interventions and the severity of cases can increase the risk of exposure to infectious agents.

1. The skin barrier :
The skin is our first line of defence against infection. It acts as a protective barrier, preventing the penetration of pathogenic micro-organisms. The integrity of this barrier must be maintained, and any injury or cut must be treated immediately.
2. Personal protective equipment (PPE) :
   Gloves: They must be worn whenever there is contact with blood, body fluids, mucous membranes or non-intact skin. They must be changed between each patient.
   Masks and respirators: These reduce the risk of inhaling infectious agents. The choice of surgical mask or respirator depends on risk assessment.
   Gowns, aprons and coveralls: Protect carers from splashes of body fluids.
   Eye protection: Goggles or face shields are essential where splashes are a possibility.

3. Hand hygiene :
One of the most effective ways of preventing transmission is regular and thorough hand washing with soap and water or the use of alcohol-based disinfectants. Hands should be washed before and after each interaction with a patient, after removing PPE, after using the toilet and before eating.

4. Respiratory label :
Coughing or sneezing into a tissue or your elbow, avoiding touching your face, and washing your hands immediately after coughing or sneezing help prevent the spread of respiratory infections.

5. Handling and disposal of medical waste :
Potentially contaminated medical waste must be handled with care and disposed of in accordance with health guidelines.

6. Cleaning and disinfection :
Surfaces, especially those that are frequently touched, must be regularly cleaned and disinfected. Medical instruments must be properly sterilised.

7. Training and awareness :
Regular staff training on the correct use of PPE, hand hygiene and prevention procedures is essential.

8. Vaccination :
Vaccinating medical staff against common communicable diseases is another key prevention strategy.

9. Surveillance of nosocomial infections :
A surveillance system must be put in place to rapidly identify any outbreaks of infection within the establishment and take appropriate action.

Personal protection and the prevention of transmission are fundamental elements of medical practice. By putting in place rigorous measures and ensuring that they are adhered to, healthcare establishments can protect both medical staff and patients, while ensuring the highest quality of care.

Psychological support for patients, families and staff

The urgent and often unexpected nature of acute medicine generates a high level of stress not only for patients, but also for their families and nursing staff. Managing this pressure requires a solid infrastructure of psychological support.

1. For patients :

Emotional support: On arrival, patients are often overwhelmed by fear and anxiety. Establishing a relationship of trust, being available to listen and sharing clear information can alleviate these feelings.

Pain management: In addition to physical pain, patients can also experience emotional pain. Holistic pain assessment and tailored interventions can offer real relief.

Availability of psychological services: Psychologists and counsellors must be easily accessible to provide appropriate support.

2. For families :

Soothing waiting rooms: These areas should be designed to provide a calm environment, with information available about patient care.

Regular updates: Transparent and regular communication with families reduces their anxiety and builds trust.

Support groups: Talking groups or workshops can help families to share their experiences and find mutual support.

3. For staff :

Supervision and support: Teams should have regular supervision sessions to discuss difficult cases, share feelings and seek solutions collectively.

Wellness programmes: Activities such as yoga, meditation or stress management workshops can be beneficial.

Access to counsellors or psychologists: Faced with traumatic situations, staff may need individual sessions.

Ongoing training: Training in communication management, conflict de-escalation or stress management can provide staff with additional tools.

Team events: Organising integration events or leisure activities can strengthen bonds within the team and provide moments of relaxation.

Psychological support in acute medicine is an essential pillar in guaranteeing the quality of care and well-being of all. Medical institutions, aware of the emotional and psychological impact of the acute environment, must put in place robust support mechanisms for patients, their families and staff.

Chapter 26.
ADVANCES AND RESEARCH
IN ACUTE MEDICINE

Latest discoveries
and advances in acute care

The world of medicine is constantly evolving, and acute medicine is no exception. Thanks to technological advances, new research and improved protocols, the field of acute care is undergoing constant transformation to improve the quality of care offered to patients.

1. Advanced medical imaging technologies :
Advances in imaging, such as point-of-care ultrasound and faster scans, allow clinicians to diagnose more accurately and quickly, reducing the time needed to administer appropriate treatment.

2. Artificial intelligence and data analysis :
AI is increasingly being used to anticipate potential complications in patients, by analysing complex data in real time. This improves the efficiency of care and the prevention of critical situations.

3. Telemedicine :
Although telemedicine was already on the increase, the COVID-19 pandemic has boosted its use. It enables remote assessment, which is essential for remote regions or when acute care units are overloaded.

4. Targeted therapies and personalised medicine :
Understanding the molecular and genetic mechanisms of diseases has led to the development of more targeted

therapies. Treatments can now be tailored to the patient's genetics, improving efficacy and reducing side effects.

5. New drugs and treatments :
Pharmacological advances, such as direct anticoagulants and new antibiotics, are enriching the therapeutic arsenal of doctors in acute medicine.

6. Simulation-based training :
Simulation centres are on the increase, offering medical staff an environment in which they can train to manage emergency situations without risk to patients.

7. Improved protocols for sepsis :
Recent studies have refined management protocols for sepsis, thereby reducing the mortality associated with this condition.

8. Multidisciplinary approaches :
Integrated care, involving different specialists from the outset, is increasingly favoured to provide comprehensive and optimal care.

Advances in acute medicine are a testament to the medical field's ability to adapt and evolve in the face of new challenges. These discoveries and innovations don't just advance science; they save lives, improve patients' quality of life and boost the efficiency of medical teams. The key lies in the ongoing training of healthcare professionals to keep them at the cutting edge of these developments.

Taking part in clinical research as a nurse

Clinical research is essential for advancing medical science and improving the quality of patient care. Nurses, who are at the heart of patient care, play a key role in implementing, monitoring and sometimes even designing these studies. Their active participation in clinical research brings undeniable added value.

1. The role of the nurse in clinical research :
a. Patient recruitment and consent :
Because of their close relationship with patients, nurses play a key role in recruiting them for clinical trials. They are often the first point of contact for explaining the objectives, benefits and potential risks of a study, and for obtaining informed consent.
b. Data collection :
The nurse is responsible for the regular and accurate collection of clinical data. This may include taking vital signs, collecting biological samples or documenting side effects.
c. Treatment administration :
In drug trials, the nurse is often responsible for administering the treatment, whether it's a new drug or a new dosage.
d. Evaluation and monitoring :
The nurse monitors patients throughout the study, evaluating their response to treatment and monitoring any side effects.
e. Education and communication :
The nurse educates patients about the study protocols, answers their questions and acts as a liaison between the patient and the research team.

2. Advantages for the nurse :
a. Professional development :
Taking part in clinical research offers a unique opportunity to learn about the latest medical advances and acquire new skills.
b. Contribution to science :

By taking part in research, nurses contribute directly to improving care and advancing medical science.

c. Diversity of role :

Clinical research can offer a welcome change from the usual routines, with new challenges and responsibilities.

3. The challenges :

a. Ethics :

Nurses must always ensure that patients' rights and safety are respected, in accordance with the ethical principles of research.

b. Workload :

Research can add an extra layer of responsibility, requiring effective management of time and priorities.

c. Continuing training :

Clinical research is a constantly evolving field, requiring knowledge to be updated on a regular basis.

Nurses, through their proximity to patients, clinical expertise and dedication, are key players in clinical research. Although this can present challenges, the positive impact on the quality of care, the opportunity for professional development and the contribution to science make it a rewarding experience.

Integrating new practices in routine care

Over the years, advances in medical research, technological developments and feedback have led to the emergence of new healthcare practices. These new methodologies, when properly integrated, can improve the effectiveness of treatments, the quality of care, and even the well-being of patients and healthcare professionals. But how are these new practices adopted and integrated into routine care?

1. Evaluation of new practices :

a. Scientific validation :

Before being widely adopted, any new practice must undergo rigorous evaluation, often through clinical trials, to ensure its effectiveness and safety.

b. Comparison with current practices :

It is essential to compare the new approach with existing methods to determine whether it offers a real improvement.

2. Training and education :

a. Continuing training :

Healthcare professionals, such as doctors, nurses and technicians, need to be trained in the new methods. This often involves workshops, seminars and practical training sessions.

b. Raising awareness :

It is also crucial to inform patients and their families, where relevant, about new methods and what they can expect.

3. Gradual implementation :

a. Drivers and test programs :

Before widespread adoption, new practices can be tested in a controlled environment, for example in a particular department or hospital.

b. Feedback :

The first uses will provide feedback that will be essential for refining and adjusting the practice.

4. Adapting infrastructures :

a. Equipment and technology :

If a new practice requires the use of new technologies or equipment, it will be crucial to ensure that medical facilities are equipped accordingly.

b. Protocols and guidelines :

Standard medical protocols and guidelines may need to be updated to incorporate the new method.

5. Continuous assessment :

a. Monitoring results :

Even after adopting a new practice, it is essential to continue monitoring and evaluating its results to ensure that it continues to benefit patients.

b. Adaptability :

Healthcare professionals must remain flexible and ready to adjust or modify practice if necessary, depending on results or new information.

Integrating new practices into routine care is a complex process requiring careful evaluation, appropriate training and careful implementation. However, with a commitment to clinical excellence and patient wellbeing, these innovations can lead to better care and improved patient outcomes.

Chapter 27.
CAREER DEVELOPMENT
AND CONTINUING EDUCATION

Specialisations in acute medicine

Acute medicine is a broad field that encompasses the management of patients with sudden, often life-threatening conditions. Although acute medicine itself is a speciality, it comprises a number of sub-specialities depending on the specific needs of patients and the skills required to treat them. These sub-specialties require additional training and specific expertise to ensure optimal patient care.

1. Emergency medicine
Emergency medicine focuses on the immediate assessment and treatment of patients presenting to emergency departments. This requires skills in triage, rapid diagnosis and treatment of a wide range of conditions.

2. Medical resuscitation
Intensive care doctors work in intensive care units, treating the most seriously ill or injured patients. They manage complex cases requiring continuous monitoring and intervention.

3. Acute interventional cardiology
This sub-field deals with cardiac emergencies, such as myocardial infarction, using interventional techniques to restore blood flow.

4. Emergency neurology
Emergency neurologists specialise in treating emergencies such as strokes, haemorrhages and brain injuries.

5. Traumatology
Traumatologists treat serious injuries resulting from accidents, falls or violence. This can include complex fractures, internal injuries and multiple traumas.

6. Emergency paediatrics
Emergency paediatrics focuses on the management of medical emergencies in children, from newborns to adolescents.

7. Emergency toxicology
This speciality deals with poisoning, overdoses and exposure to dangerous substances, often requiring rapid intervention to prevent damage or death.

8. Obstetric and gynaecological emergencies
Specialising in emergencies relating to pregnancy, childbirth and gynaecological conditions.

9. Emergency psychiatry
Management of acute psychiatric crises, such as psychotic episodes, suicide attempts or mental health emergencies.

10. Acute geriatric medicine
Focused on the unique needs of elderly patients who may present with atypical symptoms and have multiple co-morbidities.

Acute medicine, by its very nature, demands rapid action, precise decision-making and specific expertise. The sub-specialties mentioned above provide a more focused and specialised approach to dealing with the various medical emergencies. As medicine and technology continue to develop, it is likely that new sub-specialties will emerge to meet the changing needs of the population.

Importance of continuing training

In the ever-changing world of health and medicine, continuing education plays a key role in ensuring the delivery of high-quality, safe and effective care. Continuing education is not only a regulatory requirement for many healthcare professionals, it is also fundamental to their professional and personal development. Here's why continuing education is so important:

1. Updating knowledge
Medical research is evolving at a rapid pace. New studies, techniques, protocols and medicines are constantly emerging. Continuing education enables healthcare professionals to keep abreast of the latest advances, ensuring that patients benefit from the latest and most effective treatments.

2. Skills enhancement
As well as acquiring new knowledge, continuing education offers the opportunity to perfect existing skills and learn new ones, whether clinical, administrative or interpersonal.

3. Improving patient safety
Medical errors can have serious consequences. Regular training in best practice, safety protocols and the appropriate use of equipment can reduce the risk of errors and improve patient safety.

4. Meeting regulatory requirements
Many regulatory bodies require healthcare professionals to undergo a certain amount of continuing education in order to maintain their licence or certification. This guarantees a minimum standard of training and competence.

5. Professional development

Continuing education can open the door to new specialities, career advancement or leadership roles. It's also an opportunity for networking, exchanging ideas with colleagues and learning from others.

6. Increased trust

By staying informed and improving their skills, healthcare professionals gain confidence in their ability to provide quality care.

7. Meeting society's changing needs

Continuing training enables healthcare professionals to adapt to demographic changes, new pathologies and health crises such as pandemics.

8. Promoting interdisciplinarity

Training courses can often be multidisciplinary, offering the opportunity to learn how other professions approach care, thereby promoting more effective collaboration.

9. Renewed passion and commitment

Continuing education can rekindle passion for the profession, offer a break from the daily grind and remind professionals why they chose their vocation.

10. Ethical responsibility

Healthcare professionals have an ethical duty to provide the best possible care. Continuing education is one way of honouring this commitment by ensuring that their skills and knowledge are up to date.

Continuing education is much more than just an obligation or a box to tick. It's a commitment to professional excellence, patient safety and quality of care. In a field as vital and dynamic as healthcare, continuing education is the pillar that underpins competence, confidence and compassion.

Participating in research and innovation

The world of acute medicine, like many other areas of healthcare, is profoundly influenced by advances in research and innovation. These elements do more than simply guide treatments or protocols: they constantly redefine what is possible in terms of patient care. Active participation in research and innovation is essential for any professional wishing not only to maintain but also to improve the quality of the care they provide. Here's why and how to get involved:

1. Staying at the cutting edge of knowledge
Medical research is constantly evolving. By becoming actively involved, healthcare professionals can keep abreast of the latest discoveries, techniques and approaches, enabling them to provide care based on the most up-to-date evidence.

2. Contribute to the advancement of medicine
Taking part in research gives you the opportunity to be at the forefront of the discoveries that will shape the medicine of tomorrow. It's a chance to contribute directly to improving treatments and interventions that will benefit generations of patients.

3. Developing expertise
Involvement in research or innovation projects enables you to specialise in specific areas, acquire new skills and become a benchmark in your field.

4. Interdisciplinary collaboration
Medical research and innovation are often the result of interdisciplinary collaboration. This provides an opportunity to exchange ideas with experts in other fields, to learn from their perspectives and to bring a richer, more complete dimension to projects.

5. Meeting unmet needs
Participation in research helps to identify and respond to unmet medical needs, whether in terms of treatments, devices, techniques or procedures.

6. Facilitating the adoption of new practices
Those involved in research and innovation are often the first to adopt and promote new practices, playing an essential role in training their colleagues and implementing beneficial changes.

7. Institutional support and funding
Many institutions encourage research by offering funding, training or resources. Taking an active part can open up funding opportunities for projects, conferences or training courses.

8. Professional recognition
The contribution made to research and innovation is often recognised and valued, offering visibility and recognition at national or international level.

9. Ethics and responsibility
It is the duty of healthcare professionals to constantly seek to improve patient care. Research and innovation are direct means of fulfilling this ethical imperative.

Research and innovation in acute medicine are essential to advancing medicine and improving patient care. By becoming actively involved, healthcare professionals play a direct role in shaping the future of their field, while developing professionally and enriching their practices.

Chapter 28.
THE FUTURE OF ACUTE MEDICINE

Emerging trends and future challenges

Acute medicine, at the intersection of technology, research and clinical needs, is constantly evolving. Emerging trends are shaping the current landscape and posing new challenges for the future. Here is an exploration of some of these trends and the obstacles they may present.

1. Artificial Intelligence (AI) and Machine Learning

With the rise of AI, advanced algorithms can now aid diagnosis, predict clinical outcomes and personalise care. While this has revolutionary potential, it also raises questions about data security, ethics and dependence on technology.

2. Telemedicine

The COVID-19 pandemic has brought telemedicine to the forefront. While telemedicine offers greater flexibility and accessibility, it also poses challenges in terms of confidentiality, equipment and staff training.

3. Antibiotic resistance

The excessive and inappropriate use of antibiotics has led to an increase in resistant bacteria, making certain infections more difficult to treat. This is a major challenge for acute medicine, requiring careful and educational management of prescriptions.

4. Changing demographics

With an ageing population in many parts of the world, hospitals and clinics are faced with an increase in chronic diseases and co-morbidities. This calls for a multidisciplinary approach and specific training.

5. Personalised care

Personalised medicine, based on the patient's genetics and biomedical data, is gaining ground. While this promises more targeted treatments, it also implies in-depth training and equitable access to resources.

6. Health crises and pandemics

The ability to respond rapidly to epidemics or pandemics is essential. Recent crises have shown the importance of preparation, training and flexibility in responding to health emergencies.

7. Professional burnout

Stress and pressure in acute medicine have led to high rates of burnout. It is crucial to put in place support, training and welfare measures for staff.

8. Innovations in equipment

New, more portable and connected medical devices are making it easier to monitor and treat patients. However, these innovations mean that staff skills need to be constantly updated.

9. Continuing training

With the rapid evolution of medicine, the need for continuing education and specialisation is more pressing than ever to ensure quality care.

10. Ethical issues

Ethical dilemmas such as informed consent, the end of life and access to care remain at the heart of medical practice and require constant reflection.

As acute medicine adapts and evolves in the face of these trends and challenges, it continues to be a dynamic field that requires constant monitoring, adaptability and a commitment to clinical excellence. By staying informed and collaborating on a global scale, healthcare professionals can overcome these challenges and deliver quality care to all patients.

Technology and telemedicine :
What is the impact?

Technology, with its rapid and relentless evolution, has revolutionised almost every aspect of our daily lives. In medicine, and particularly in telemedicine, these changes are profound and transformative. Let's explore the impact of technology and telemedicine on modern medicine.

1. Improved access to care
Telemedicine breaks down geographical barriers, providing access to healthcare for people who are remote, isolated or have reduced mobility. This means that a patient living in a remote area can consult a specialist without having to travel long distances.

2. Cost reduction
The ability to consult remotely can reduce the costs associated with travel, unnecessary hospitalisation and excessive use of emergency services.

3. Ongoing monitoring
With connected devices, doctors can remotely monitor patients' vital signs and state of health, which is particularly beneficial for those suffering from chronic illnesses.

4. Efficiency and time savings
Telemedicine can reduce waiting times and make it easier to book appointments, thereby improving the efficiency of the healthcare system.

5. Patient education and empowerment
Telemedicine platforms often offer educational resources, enabling patients to better understand their condition and actively participate in their care.

6. Confidentiality and security challenges
With the digitisation of medical records and online consultations, the protection of patient data is becoming paramount. Platforms must guarantee flawless security to prevent data breaches.

7. Quality of care

While telemedicine offers many benefits, quality of care is a concern. Can remote consultation really replace face-to-face interaction? It depends on the situation, but it's an ongoing debate.

8. Training and regulations

The introduction of technology into medicine requires healthcare professionals to be trained in the new tools and platforms. In addition, regulations must evolve to adapt to this new form of medical practice.

9. Evolution of care models

With telemedicine, the traditional model of the patient coming to the hospital or clinic is changing. We are moving towards a model where care comes to the patient, wherever he or she may be.

10. Technological barriers

Not everyone has access to the technology needed for telemedicine or is comfortable using it. It is crucial to ensure that these innovations benefit everyone, not just a technological elite.

Technology and telemedicine are redefining medicine as we know it. While they offer unparalleled opportunities to improve care and efficiency, they also present challenges that need to be approached with caution and foresight. The future of medicine will undoubtedly be shaped by these innovations, and it is essential to ensure that they are used ethically and fairly.

The changing role of the nurse in a changing world

In the vast world of healthcare, nurses are the pillars who, often behind the scenes, guarantee continuity of care and patient safety. With technological advances, socio-cultural upheavals and successive health crises, the role of the nurse is constantly evolving. Let's take a closer look at this profound and necessary transformation.

1. The nurse, beyond technical care
Whereas in the past, nurses were seen primarily as executors of medical prescriptions, today they are recognised as true clinicians. They assess, plan and implement interventions and evaluate their effectiveness. This expanded role stems in part from the recognition of clinical skills and the need for a holistic approach to care.

2. Specialised expertise
Medical advances and the growing needs of the population have led to the emergence of a wide range of nursing specialities: anaesthetists, neonatal nurses, oncology nurses, cardiology nurses, etc. These specialities require additional training and make it possible to offer high-precision care. These specialities require additional training and make it possible to offer high-precision care.

3. The nurse practitioner
Some countries have introduced the role of the nurse practitioner, who has advanced training and can prescribe medicines, make diagnoses or initiate treatment. This helps to lighten the burden on doctors and improve access to care.

4. Technology and nursing care
Digitalisation is also having an impact on the nursing profession. From electronic medical records to remote monitoring tools, nurses must adapt to these new methods, while ensuring that humanity remains at the heart of their practice.

5. Health promotion and prevention
Today's nurse plays a crucial role in preventing disease and promoting healthy lifestyles. This educational role is essential in the face of today's public health challenges.

6. Change agent
Nurses are increasingly involved in quality improvement initiatives, helping to shape the future of healthcare systems through research, education and advocacy.

7. Societal challenges and health crises
Emergencies such as the COVID-19 pandemic have highlighted the flexibility, resilience and crucial importance of nurses. Faced with the unknown, they were on the front line, adapting their practices, managing risks and supporting patients at extremely difficult times.

8. Ethical issues
With the growing complexity of care and the moral dilemmas associated with the end of life, medical innovation and health equity, nurses are often faced with situations that require in-depth ethical reflection.

The evolving role of nurses reflects the changing dynamics of our society and the ever-growing needs of healthcare systems. These professionals, with their dedication and expertise, will continue to be key players, adapting and innovating to meet the challenges of tomorrow. While the world changes, the heart of nursing - the commitment to the well-being and dignity of the patient - remains constant.

Chapter 29.
RESOURCES AND TOOLS FOR NURSES IN ACUTE MEDICINE

Books, journals and key publications

In acute medicine and nursing, there is a wealth of valuable resources for professionals who want to expand their knowledge and keep abreast of the latest advances and best practice. Here is a non-exhaustive list of key books, journals and publications that are particularly relevant to these fields:

Books :

- **"Emergency Nursing: Principles and Practice** by Gary Jones and Ruth Endacott - A comprehensive guide for nurses working in the emergency services.
- **"Critical Care Nursing: Diagnosis and Management** by Linda D. Urden, Kathleen M. Stacy, and Mary E. Lough - A must-have reference for critical care.
- **"Pediatric Emergency Medicine"** by Gary R. Strange and Robert W. Schafermeyer - For those who work with children in emergency settings.
- **"Advanced Practice Nursing in the Care of Older Adults"** by Laurie Kennedy-Malone, Kathleen Ryan Fletcher, and Lori Martin-Plank - Focused on gerontology and care of the elderly.

Newspapers :

- **Journal of Emergency Nursing (JEN)**: The official publication of the Emergency Nurses Association (ENA), it covers topics relevant to emergency nurses.

Critical Care Nurse (CCN): A journal dedicated to critical care nurses, offering research articles, case studies and literature reviews.

American Journal of Critical Care (AJCC): Publishes research, commentary and practical articles for critical care professionals.

Pediatric Emergency Care: Focusing on paediatric emergencies, this is an essential resource for those working with younger patients.

Key publications :

"Guidelines for the Management of Acute Care Patients: A publication frequently updated by various professional associations, providing evidence-based guidelines for the management of patients in acute situations.

"Standards of Critical Care Nursing Practice: Sets standards for nurses practising in intensive care units.

"Emergency Triage: Manchester Triage Group: An essential manual for triage in the emergency services, widely adopted internationally.

It is important to note that the relevance of these resources may vary according to region, country and local protocols. In addition, with the rapid evolution of medicine and healthcare practices, it is crucial for healthcare professionals to regularly consult updated sources and participate in continuing education.

Here is a non-exhaustive list of relevant resources for French-speaking professionals:

Books :

"Urgences pour l'infirmier" by S. David - A practical and comprehensive guide for nurses dealing with emergency situations.

"Nursing practice in intensive care" by C. Dupont and C. Aubert - This book offers a comprehensive approach to care in intensive care units.

"Urgences pédiatriques" by V. Gajdos and B. Chevallier - A reference for the management of emergencies in children.

"Soins palliatifs: guide pratique pour les professionnels de la santé" by B. Rioualen and P. Grandet - An essential resource on end-of-life care.

Newspapers :

"Revue de l'Infirmière": a journal covering professional news, innovations in care and the challenges facing the profession.

"Soins; la revue de référence infirmière" : Covers a variety of topics relevant to nurses, with a particular focus on clinical practice.

"Annales Françaises de Médecine d'Urgence": A publication focusing on emergency medicine in France, including research articles, reviews and case studies.

"Réanimation": Journal dedicated to intensive care and resuscitation.

Key publications :

"Recommendations for Clinical Practice (RPC): Published by various learned societies, these recommendations provide evidence-based guidelines for various clinical situations.

"Protocols in obstetric anaesthesia and analgesia": A key publication for those working in the field of anaesthesia, particularly in obstetrics.

"Guide de triage aux urgences": Based on the Canadian Emergency Triage and Acuity System (CTAS), this guide is widely used in French-speaking emergency departments.

It is essential for French-speaking healthcare professionals to keep up to date with the latest advances in their field. This means regularly consulting relevant publications, attending training courses and conferences, and getting involved in professional networks.

Professional associations and networking

Networking and membership of professional associations are essential for nurses and other healthcare professionals. They provide opportunities for professional development, knowledge exchange, continuing education, and professional and emotional support. For French-speaking professionals, there are many relevant associations:

1. General professional associations :
   - **Ordre National des Infirmiers (ONI):** This is the umbrella organisation for nurses in France. Its aim is to represent the profession, defend its interests and offer resources to professionals.
   - **Fédération Interprofessionnelle de la Santé du Québec (FIQ)**: This Quebec organisation mainly represents nurses and nursing assistants.
2. Specialist professional associations :
   - **Société Française de Médecine d'Urgence (SFMU) (French Society for Emergency Medicine):** brings together professionals working in the field of medical emergencies and promotes research, education and training in this sector.
   - Association Française de Pédiatrie Ambulatoire (AFPA): For those specialising in paediatrics.
   - **Société de Réanimation de Langue Française (SRLF) (French-language resuscitation society):** This concerns professionals working in resuscitation departments.
3. Networking groups :
   - **The Journées Internationales de la Qualité Hospitalière et en Santé (JIQHS): This is an** annual event for healthcare professionals wishing to discuss quality of care and patient safety.

Nurses' congresses: Various congresses are held on a regular basis to provide an opportunity for training and networking.

4. Online platforms :

Infirmiers.com: This is an information portal and forum for French-speaking nurses.

Professional social networks such as LinkedIn also allow you to connect with colleagues, participate in specialist groups and keep up to date with the latest news and opportunities in your field.

Nurses and other healthcare professionals are advised to join one or more of these associations and take an active part in their activities. Not only can this enrich their professional careers, but it can also offer them valuable support, particularly in areas as demanding as acute medicine.

Courses and training, and additional certifications

In the field of acute medicine, it is imperative that nurses and other healthcare professionals continue their education and training throughout their careers. This not only ensures that their skills are constantly updated, but also meets the changing demands of technology, techniques and clinical guidelines. Here are some of the courses, training and further qualifications relevant to nurses in this field:

1. Emergency training :
   - **Advanced Life Support (ALS)**: advanced training in cardiopulmonary resuscitation.
   - **Pediatric Advanced Life Support (PALS)**: Focuses on paediatric emergencies.
   - **Trauma Nursing Core Course (TNCC)**: Specific to nursing care for trauma patients.
2. Medical specialities :
   - **Certification in intensive care** : For those who work or wish to work in intensive care.
   - **Cardiology certification**: Specific to acute cardiac care.
3. Management of specific patients :
   - **Emergency mental health training: Managing** psychiatric crises in emergency settings.
   - **Training in geriatrics**: Specific to the management of elderly patients in emergency situations.
4. Additional training :
   - **Certification in crisis management**: Essential for managing situations such as violence or aggression in the hospital environment.
   - **Training in medical communication**: to improve communication with patients, their families and the healthcare team.

5. Technology and equipment :

- **Certification in emergency ultrasound**: Use of ultrasound for rapid diagnosis in emergency situations.
- **Telemedicine training**: for the use of remote communication technologies in patient care.

6. Management and leadership :

- **Team management training**: For head nurses or those aspiring to leadership roles.
- **Medical ethics course**: Navigating complex ethical situations in acute medicine.

7. Research training :

- **Research methodology course**: For nurses interested in clinical or academic research.

It should be noted that the availability and relevance of these courses and certifications can vary from region to region and from country to country. In addition, attending conferences, workshops and seminars is also an excellent way of keeping abreast of the latest trends and advances in the field.